Fighting Solves Everything:

Destroying Cancer with Faith, Nutrition, and Science

By
Paul G. Markel

Fighting Solves Everything:

Destroying Cancer with Faith, Nutrition, and Science

By
Paul G. Markel

Paul G. Markel © 2019

No part of this text may be reproduced without the express written permission of the author and publisher.

Dedication

Throughout my fight against cancer, there have been a great number of people who have helped me and given me support. Throughout the following pages I plan to thank and appreciate these people.

However, this book would never have been finished, and I have doubts about whether I would still be here and in the shape I am, without the tireless and selfless love and care that I received from Nancy, my wife. She is my compass and my strength.

At first we cried together. Then we fought together. Nancy stayed by my side through the pain and sickness and my inability to eat or drink. She spent hours in the kitchen preparing special meals for me and then fed me through a tube in my stomach.

Nancy was patient with me when I was tired and grumpy and downright unpleasant to be around. She went with me to every doctor's appointment and lab test. She spent countless hours sitting in a waiting room while I was in the back being poked with needles, scanned, and irradiated.

My beloved bride read hundreds of articles online about the Keto diet, natural cancer treatments, nutrition, pain medication, and what to expect when someone has the type of cancer I had. She kept up with my myriad appointments with doctors, therapists, and lab tests.

I've expressed most of the above to my close friends and one of them put it best when he said; "You married well." Indeed, I did.

A wife of noble character who can find? She is worth far more than rubies. Proverbs 31:10

Contents

Dedication   4

Introduction   7

Chapter 1   Dealing with the Big Black
              Question Mark 9

Chapter 2   The Move   21
Chapter 3   Keto Diet   24
Chapter 4   Barbell Training   31
Chapter 5   Treatment   36
Chapter 6   The Study   45
Chapter 7   Hospitalized   50
Chapter 8   Nutrition   61
Chapter 9   Faith   66
Chapter 10   Avoiding the Victim Mentality   71
Chapter 11   Support Network   76
Chapter 12   The Recovery   78
Chapter 13   The Results   87
Chapter 14   The Moral of the Story   90

Bonus Material
Nancy's Story   92
Good Food Recipes   113

Introduction

This will be the most difficult book for me to ever write. For the last twenty plus years, when I needed or wanted to write a book, I opened up a document and just started writing. I already knew in my head what I wanted to say and what I wanted to impart to the reader. This time is different. For the most part, I have always known how the book that I was writing would end.

What I am about to write is not something about which I had ever planned or intended. All things being equal, I would rather not have this experience or be able to share this with others. Nonetheless, in this life, we don't get to make some decisions; they are made for us and it is up to us to deal with the situations in which we find ourselves.

From nearly the moment I received my cancer diagnosis, I felt that this challenge was put before me for a reason. I have a strong faith in God and truly believe that He will never give me more than I can handle.

Before I began typing, I had several internal discussions. As you would expect, I experienced the full battery of emotions. "Why me?" "This is not supposed to happen to me." "What am I going to do now?"

One of the biggest struggles was, do I tell anyone other than my immediate family? The hard headed man in me said "keep it to yourself" and "don't burden other people with your problems".

I have had the great fortune in my life to have several honest, genuine, and faithful friends. After a few conversations with those friends, I understood that I not only had the opportunity to use this personal difficulty/challenge to help others, I had an obligation. I have an obligation to use this test, and my experience during it, to provide inspiration, motivation, and assistance to others who may be going through a similar situation or have loved ones who are as well.

A word of caution, you may encounter some adult language/cuss words in the pages that follow. There are a few rules when you beat cancer. One of them is; when you beat cancer you get to eat pizza and/or donuts. Another rule is; when you beat cancer you get to use whatever words you choose, including cuss words. Those are the rules, deal with them.

So that's it, short and sweet. An introduction that was actually written before I had any idea of what the ending would be.

PGM 4/2/19

Dealing with the Big, Black Question Mark

When I discovered a lump on the right side of my neck, I thought it was a swollen lymph node. Dr. Google told me that a lymph node will swell if you have been exposed to a virus or bacteria. Dr. Google also said that the swelling would normally go away within two weeks. If not, go see a real doctor.

Well, the swelling did not go away after two weeks, so I made my first appointment with a family doctor. The GP (General Practitioner) Dr. Susan Foley, ruled out lymph node and opined that the swelling was my salivary gland. Apparently, salivary glands can develop stones and become blocked.

Living in a small mountain town, such as Saratoga, Wyoming, is wonderful. Small community, no traffic, beautiful scenery. However, for serious medical treatment, you need to travel. My first trip was to Rawlins, Wyoming for an Ultrasound of the lump. That wasn't so bad, under an hour travel time (one way).

Five days later the results of the test were determined to be "inconclusive". We needed another test, this time a CT scan with contrast. Book the appointment. Travel back to Rawlins. Wait another week.

Now the results are "abnormal cell activity". We need to send you to an Ear, Nose, and Throat specialist for a closer look. Book that appointment and travel to Laramie, Wyoming, ninety miles, one way. We are now over two weeks into the attempt to diagnose the lump and a month since I discovered it.

The ENT guy was fantastic, Dr. Paul Johnson. During the first visit Dr. Johnson examined the lump, scoped down my nose for a closer look and removed some cells from the lump to be examined in the lab. "It's definitely a tumor and there is a 50/50 chance of it being benign or cancer."

That was a smack in the face. Tumor? It's not supposed to be a tumor. That is an old joke going back to the Kindergarten Cop movie where Schwarzenegger says "It's not a tumor." in his famous Austrian accent.

On Friday morning, February 22, 2019, I received a telephone call from Dr. Johnson. He explained that normally this conversation would take place in person but, as I was an hour and a half drive away, a call would have to do. "The tumor is cancer. Specifically, it is cystic squamous cell carcinoma." *What? What the hell is that?*

I sat down, feeling that invisible gut punch that accompanies life-altering news. "We need you to get a PET scan so we can find out exactly where the cancer is located and if it is spreading."

We decided on Cheyenne, Wyoming, 2.5 hours away, for the scanning procedure. Dr. Johnson was considerate and asked if I had questions. *Questions? Only a hundred.* We finished the call with him explaining that his nurse would contact Cheyenne Radiology and set the appointment.

There had been a question mark hanging over my head for over a month. Now the question mark was enormous and black. The lump was a tumor, the tumor was cancer. Now, where else is the cancer? Is it all in one place? Has it spread to lungs, liver, kidneys, etc? What stage is it?

The PET scan was scheduled for a week from the day of diagnosis. There was nothing to do but wait and wonder and worry and pray.

My initial reaction was to only tell my wife, Nancy, and our three kids. As fate would have it, only one son, Zach, was in Saratoga. My daughter Paxton, lived across the country in Alabama and Jarrad, my oldest was on a business trip to the west coast. That meant phone calls; shitty phone calls that you don't want to make.

What do you say? Do you just say "Hi, guess what? I have cancer?" Or, do you make small talk and then drop the cancer news as an aside? "How's the weather there? How's work going? Oh, by the way, I have cancer."

I would get some practice making those calls and I found the best way was just to get it over with at the beginning. Get the bad news out of the way as soon as possible. You can't really ease into that kind of subject.

That first week was especially difficult for my wife and life-long partner. There was a considerable amount of crying and long hugs. How did this happen? Why was it happening? My family has no history of cancer, any kind of cancer. Markel men normally die of heart-attacks in their late sixties or seventies. McClelland men, (mom's side) live long lives. My grandfather is 95 years old and living in Florida. His dad lived to 94. His brother lived to 93.

All of the grief stages began, Shock and Disbelief, this is not supposed to happen to me. It must be a bad dream. Anger and Frustration; I'm busy living my life, trying to run a business. I don't have time to be a cancer patient.

Then the heavy mortality thoughts crept in. What do I need to do if this is it? How much time do I have? What if the test results say I am "terminal"?

Many of the questions were not that difficult to answer. As for what to do with my time, the answer was to keep producing material; keep writing, keep recording radio, keep shooting video.

The day after my diagnosis, Zach, my youngest son, and I took a trip up into the mountains, to the higher elevations, to record a bunch of video material in the deep snow. I had to make the purposeful decision not to just lay down and feel sorry for myself. That's the natural human reaction and believe me, there were some long naps and times I did not want to get out of bed that first week.

Everyone likes to say "make the most of everyday, you never know when it's going to be your last". However, you don't wake up in the morning thinking, "I might be killed in a car wreck today." When you get a cancer diagnosis, you do wake up thinking, "How many days are left?" The reality of mortality is not notional, it's right in your face. That big, black question mark is a son of a bitch.

The trip to Cheyenne that week was a pleasant drive. Nancy downloaded Pink Floyd's "The Wall" onto her phone and we listened to it for the entire ride over. Thank the Lord for double albums.

Nancy had told a friend what was going on and where we were going. Her friend told her husband

and it turned out that he had had to travel to Cheyenne with his ailing mother the year before to get medical treatment for her. The gentleman walked up to Nancy at work and handed her a piece of paper. The paper had the address of a hotel and a confirmation number. He had called ahead and paid for a room so we could stay overnight; a wonderful act of kindness and it was the first of many to come.

We spent the night at The Historic Plains Hotel in downtown Cheyenne. Nancy and I enjoyed a nice meal, walked around a bit and got a good night's rest. I had to fast for a minimum of eight hours before the procedure which was set for 9 am.

The Cheyenne Radiology appointment was the first genuine "cancer patient" feeling I experienced. I was not there to find out *if* I had it, but to find out *where I had it*, besides the tumor in my neck.

For the curious, a PET scan includes an injection of radioactive glucose. Cancer cells feed on glucose and the radioactive glucose attaches to the cancer and lights up allowing the scan to detect it. The procedure begins with the injection. Then you sit in a comfortable chair and wait an hour for the contrast to get all the way through your body.

After the hour of waiting, during which I watched old "Friends" episodes on DVD, they put you in a hospital gown and have you lay on your back in the PET scan machine. It is similar to the MRI machines you have seen in movies and on TV. "We need you to hold as still as possible. If you move it will mess up the test and we will need to start over." I closed my eyes, took several settling breaths, and stayed as still as I possibly could. Twenty-eight minutes later, the technician was standing over me. "Okay, Paul you're all done." Her voice was pleasant and gentle. "You did a great job." she assured me.

Now the waiting would begin again.

Fast forward another week to another appointment with Dr. Johnson in Laramie. During this visit, Dr. Johnson confirmed that the tumor / cancer was localized, it had not spread into other parts of my body. That was a huge relief. "You have cancer, but what you have is highly treatable." Now onto the next step.

Dr. Johnson explained that in order to properly plan treatment he would need to go into my throat and remove a tissue sample for a complete biopsy. The tissue would give an idea as to the stage/severity, etc. Essentially, it was explained that the future treatment plan would be based upon what they found after the surgery to extract tissue.

As they would need to go in through my mouth and take a tissue sample from the area around the base of my tongue, I would need a general anesthetic, meaning I would be out completely for the procedure. Another week would be added to the calendar.

Even though it was a "simple procedure", all the pre-op steps still needed to be taken. No aspirin or anything like that could be taken for the week leading up to surgery. I needed to fast for a minimum of eight hours. Fortunately, the surgery was scheduled for early in the morning. I needed to be at the hospital for check-in and prep by 8 a.m.

Nancy and I drove over from Saratoga to Laramie the night before and stayed at the guest house offered by Ivinson Hospital. The guest house was very nice and comfortable and the cost was only $40. A hotel would have cost twice as much.

That last time I was put under for surgery was when I had my tonsils out in 1971. Needless to say, I don't remember that procedure. During the pre-op, the nurses asked a full battery of questions including "Do you feel safe at home?" What? Do I feel safe at home? Like from burglars? I carry a gun, I'm good.

Apparently they have to ask that question in case there is unreported abuse. I thought it was odd to ask me such a question, but like every other bureaucracy, people in medical facilities are not allowed to think for themselves; they just follow directions.

When the Anesthesiologist came into the room, he went over the procedure and what would happen. Then he went over possible side effects of the anesthesia which started with none and ended with fatality. Nothing like covering all the bases. I had a good friend of mine who died from a bad reaction to anesthesia during a "simple procedure". So, naturally I was apprehensive.

The nurse put a dose of what the Anesthesiologist called the "I don't care medicine" in my IV port and they wheeled my bed down the hallway. By the time they moved me to the surgery table, the shot had kicked in and I really didn't care. Seems the "I don't care" medicine really works. The last thing I remembered was the voice of the doctor by my head saying, "take some deep breaths for me."

I woke up coughing in the recovery room. My first thought was "the doctors are going to be mad that I'm coughing". The recovery room nurse handed me a tissue and told me to go ahead and cough. "Get it all out." she said. The world was still a bit foggy. I'm sure I said something strange, but I don't recall.

When they wheeled me back into my room, Nancy was sitting there waiting for me. Both she and the nurse had a good laugh watching and listening to me as I was coming down from the goofy anesthesia high. An hour or so later Nancy drove me home from the hospital. Now all we had to do was wait for the results of the biopsy.

The call came that Friday. Dr. Johnson's nurse explained that the lab had returned the biopsy results as "atypical cells" *Do I not have cancer after all?* Hope springs eternal. There I was, back on the emotional rollercoaster.

The answer was, I did indeed still have cancer, but a second biopsy surgery was going to be needed, just like the first one. *Seriously? Yes, seriously.* I would be right back at Ivinson Hospital, exactly one week later for the same procedure. They would squeeze me into the surgery schedule on Monday afternoon. Again, pre-op rules applied; fasting, stop taking any aspirin, etc.

On Monday morning we left Saratoga early so we had plenty of time to get to Laramie. The nurse had instructed me to check-in at 1230 for a 2 pm procedure. We arrived early, just a few minutes after noon. The OR nurse came out immediately and ushered me back into the room. A second nurse came in and they accelerated the pre-op process. They explained that the surgery team was just finishing with a patient and they wanted me ready ASAP.

Dr. Johnson came in and explained that for this procedure there would be a pathologist on hand, standing by. He, Dr. Johnson, would remove a tissue sample and pass it off to the pathologist who would examine it right there in the hospital to ensure it was a "good" cancer sample. "I'm going to keep you under until we are sure we have the sample we need" Johnson assured me. *Good, I thought, I don't want to do this a third time.* The anesthesiologist, a different guy this time, came in and delivered the same side effects speech.

True to his word, Dr. Johnson kept me out until they were sure they had a valid tissue sample. This time I was out twice as long as the previous week and Nancy was alone in the waiting room getting concerned. After another session in recovery and anaesthetic intoxication, they wheeled me back into my room where Nancy was waiting for me.

Dr. Johnson popped into the room to check on me. He assured us that they had a good sample, that it was cancer, and it would be sent to a lab for a complete analysis. His office would call after a few days with the results.

The treatment for my type of cancer would primarily be direct radiation oncology. Dr. Johnson explained that the radiation treatment was normally 7 weeks, 5 days a week. As we lived so far away from a treatment facility, Dr. Johnson asked how we planned to deal with the distance? My oldest son Jarrad, and his wife Alex, had been living in Salt Lake City, Utah for a couple of years. When we mentioned SLC as an option, Dr. Johnson responded that there was an excellent treatment facility at the University of Utah. He assured us that he could refer us there and we would be well taken care of.

Unlike the previous week, where the nurse encouraged me to take a nap and recover, checking in on me periodically, this time it seemed like they needed my room. The ER nurse hurried me through the check out procedure. She followed all of the steps, but like an impatient waitress that needs your table. It was obvious that they were ready for me to go.

I was tired and still working my way out of the sleepy drugs. Rather than make the long journey back home, we decided to just stay the night in Laramie. By the time we left the hospital it was around 5 pm and neither one of us wanted to drive 90 miles through the mountains in the dark.

The Move

Right on schedule, three days after my second biopsy surgery, I received another phone call from Dr. Johnson's office. The cancer cells had been confirmed to be a stage 2 squamous cell carcinoma. Recommend treatment would be direct radiation oncology. Dr. Johnson's nurse assured me that they would do a complete medical referral to the Huntsman Cancer Center, at the University of Utah in Salt Lake City. They would send over all of my records and test results. Now it was time to move.

After the second visit with Dr. Johnson, we understood that staying in Saratoga during the cancer treatment would be a practical impossibility. Spring snow storms could close the highway and prevent travel. The cost of fuel and the mileage on the truck would be astronomical. No, we would have to leave our beloved Saratoga and move to SLC, at least until I was well again.

As I mentioned at the outset, I do indeed have faith and believe in the favor of God. Jarrad and Alex had been living in an apartment in SLC, but just before my diagnosis they found a 4 bedroom house to rent. Four bedrooms seems big for just two people, but they thought it would be nice to have the extra space. Plus it was a house with a yard. They didn't want to pass it up.

When we knew that we would have to relocate for my cancer treatment, we had some long family discussions. Jarrad assured Nancy and I that we could move in with them until I was well again. As you would imagine, that was a huge relief. As we would learn, Salt Lake City is growing to the point where housing is at a premium. It also turned out that Jarrad's new house was only fifteen minutes from Huntsman Cancer Center.

Naturally, I wanted to get to SLC and begin my treatment as soon as possible. No one wants to let cancer just keep growing in their body. That meant packing up not only our entire house but the Student of the Gun office too. We gave ourselves an April first deadline and began the packing and moving process.

I must stress that my family worked like champs to make it all happen. Jarrad and Alex prepared everything in SLC, including securing a rental truck to be driven to Saratoga and back to SLC. Nancy got to work packing the house and Zach started packing up the office. I packed up all of my belongings, my business material, and everything else. Of course, we needed to keep working and producing SOTG radio and video material.

During this time we kept the cancer issue quiet. I decided not to tell anyone outside of the immediate family, even my parents. The reason was simple; I didn't want to call and say "I have cancer." There would be follow up questions for which I had no answers. I had not begun treatment yet, so I had no idea how I would react to it or what the doctors in SLC would have to say. So, I waited.

To the great credit of all involved, we were able to get the entire house and office packed up and ready to go by March 25. We ended up having to rent a second truck and trailer for a car. We gave away a lot of stuff to the local thrift shop and made a couple trips to the dump. I cannot express how grateful I am for the tireless effort my wife and kids put forth to make it all happen.

It was well after midnight by the time we arrived in Salt Lake City. Everyone was exhausted, but we needed to get one of the trucks unloaded because it had to be returned in the morning. After a few hours of sleep we were back at it. As you might expect, we had more stuff than one house could contain, so a whole bunch went into a storage unit. Again, everyone worked tremendously hard to get it all moved.

The Keto Diet

A sage piece of advice is that if you can get in to see an attorney the day you call them they are probably not a very good attorney. The same goes for doctors, particularly specialists. The first full day in SLC I called the number for the Huntsman Cancer Center that Dr. Johnson's office had given me. I had been referred to a Dr. Hitchcock. The nurse for Dr. Hitchcock informed me that the earliest opening they had to see her would be April 15, three weeks from the day I was calling. I accepted the appointment and thanked them.

It was disappointing that I would have to wait another 3 weeks, but there was nothing else to be done. I should point out that at the time I felt pretty good for someone with cancer growing in them. I was not in pain. I did not feel tired or sick. As a matter of fact, the lump on the right side of my throat had shrunk considerably. When I went to the doctor for the initial inspection of the lump, you could look at me and see it. It was definitely noticeable. This is a good time to discuss the ketogenic diet and the advice I received from a good friend.

As I mentioned earlier, when I received the "you have cancer" phone call in February, Jarrad, my oldest son, was on a business trip. He was visiting with our friend and associate, Dr. Dan Olesnicky of

SWAT Fuel. Dr. Dan is an ER doctor, as well as a certified nutritionist. Dan also co-authored a book on stem cell replacement therapy.

About fifteen minutes after I got off the phone with Jarrad, my phone rang again. It was Jarrad's number. He said, "Dad, Dan wants to talk to you." and he handed the phone to Dr. Dan. Dan had already done his own research on squamous cell carcinoma and said that, with the right treatment there was an 85-90 percent survival rate. He went on to assure me that at my age and with my current health condition, there was no reason we could not bump that up to 95 percent.

"I want you to get on the Keto diet right away." Dr. Dan told me and went on to explain. "In layman's terms, cancer cells feed on sugar. Artificial sweeteners (Sucralose, Aspartame, etc) are even worse. They are like 'miracle grow' for cancer cells" The ketogenic diet forces a metabolic change in your body and, rather than burning sugar for energy, your body burns fat and protein for energy. Yes, I understand that scientifically it is more complex than that, but that was all the information I needed.

On February 24, 2019, I started the Keto diet and I stuck to it 100 percent until I was hospitalized, but that is getting ahead of the story.

To give you an idea of what the Keto diet entails, for my age, sex, and weight, I needed to consume no more than 30 grams of carbohydrates or 5 percent of my total food intake per day. The average person takes in nearly 50 percent of their daily food in carbohydrates. Carbohydrates are not just sugar, they are anything that the body converts to sugar; grains, potatoes, fruit, dairy products, etc. If you decide to go Keto, you might be shocked at what foods are carbs and how many carbs are in what you eat.

Dr. Dan was the first medical professional to advise the Keto diet, but not the last. During this process I also had my annual physical. Dr. Foley, the GP, reviewed my blood work and physical results. With the exception of having cancer, I was in good shape for a 51 year old man. When I told her that my friend Dr. Dan had advised Keto she responded, "Good, I was going to tell you to do that, but since you already are, keep it up."

During a follow up visit with Dr. Johnson in Laramie, he expressed the same sentiment as Dr. Foley did. Now I really felt committed to the Keto diet, not that I didn't before, but it made me feel psychologically better. It made me feel like I was doing something proactive and positive to fight the cancer in my body. It gave me a small sense of control. So, for at least six weeks before I had my first consult at Huntsman, I was on the Keto diet.

About that time I talked to my friend, Jeff Kirkham, owner of Readyman and inventor of the RATS tourniquet. Jeff told me that his brother-in-law was a cancer research specialist. Several years before, Jeff's brother-in-law had asked him to be a control subject for research he was doing on, you guessed it, the effects of the ketogenic diet on patients undergoing cancer treatment. The upshot of the study was that patients who maintained a strict Keto diet showed a 50 percent higher success rate in beating cancer than those who just ate a standard diet.

The title of the study is **Using Ketogenic Diets to Enhance Radio-Chemo-Therapy Response** the author (Jeff's brother-in-law) **Bryan G Allen, MD PhD,** Division of Free Radical and Radiation Biology, Department of Radiation Oncology, University of Iowa Hospitals and Clinics, 11/4/10. Please type that into a search engine and read the study for yourself.

Now, I did not stay at a Holiday Inn Express last night, but all of the advice and information I received seemed pretty convincing that I should keep up with the ketogenic diet.

When I had my last appointment with Dr. Johnson in Laramie, the week before moving to SLC, he remarked that the lump in my neck was decidedly smaller. The lump was still detectable to the touch, but you could no longer see it when you looked at me. I took that as a good sign.

If the Keto diet is such a good thing, why isn't every cancer patient doing it? There are two primary reasons; first the gallows mentality that creeps into the human brain; "If I'm going to die, I'm going to enjoy myself and eat anything I want." Eating keto is tough. You have to make a serious, hard change to your eating habits and most humans do not possess the strength of character to make that change. Why do you think the weight loss industry is a Billion Dollar a year industry? Companies make millions by convincing people that they have a miracle shake or miracle workout machine that burns away fat with little to no commitment on the part of the user. That's all bullshit and we should know better. Regardless, people keep looking for a miracle diet or miracle machine. They don't exist.

The second reason that all cancer patients are not on keto is plain old institutionalized stubbornness or stupidity, take your pick. If a cancer doctor did not learn about keto in their formal schooling and it is not part of their clinically approved method, they will either not know about it or if they do hear about it, they will dismiss it out of hand.

You might have encountered this as the "Not Invented Here Syndrome". I have been dealing with the NIHS all my professional life as a trainer and instructor. Often it does not matter that something new is superior or beneficial, if it is not in the approved material (3 Ring Binder) it is ignored or even attacked. This is what I discovered the first day I walked into the Huntsman Cancer Center.

Now, the Huntsman Cancer Center has a terrific reputation. Nancy did a lot of research before we moved to SLC. Huntsman is highly respected for what they do and they have a great success rate for curing cancer. My words, not theirs. I would discover that cancer doctors never use the words "heal" or "cure". They say "remission" or "positive diagnosis" or "clean scan". Don't believe me? Try to get a cancer doctor to say they will cure you. I have talked to more than my share and not one has ever said "cure" or "heal".

Back to the Keto part of the story. When I met with Dr. Ying Hitchcock on April 15th, 2019, I was feeling pretty upbeat. Like I said, I was not feeling sick or in pain. I had been on Keto for six weeks and the lump in my neck was definitely smaller than when this all started. I said to her, "I am going to be one of the success stories you tell other patients about." I told her I was doing the Keto diet and expected to be praised as I had been before. Instead she immediately dismissed it. "You don't need to lose weight." she said. "You need to keep your weight and trust the treatment we will give you."

I knew right then that she did not get it and that she was not at all aware of Dr. Bryan Allen's study on Keto and cancer treatment. This reaction would prove to be the typical one I would get from all the other doctors that I consulted with at Huntsman. The staff dietician that we met with dismissed the Keto diet as a fad and suggested that in order to keep my weight on I should eat lots of potatoes and even tofu. Yes, tofu (soybean curd).

It got to the point where I just stopped talking about the Keto diet. That information was obviously not in their prescribed playbook, therefore it was not valid or even to be considered.

Having faith in our friends, Dan and Jeff, and what we had learned about Keto and cancer treatment, Nancy and I decided to keep right on doing what we were doing. I should note that I really did not lose all that much weight during the pre-treatment phase. I started at right around 245 pounds. When I began my radiation treatment the beginning of May, I weighed about 237 or 238 pounds. I don't remember exactly, but that's close.

Barbell Training

I met Matt Reynolds through my good friend James Yeager while I still lived in Biloxi, Mississippi. James had convinced Matt, a former professional strongman and nationally respected strength trainer to come to Camden, Tennessee and put on a two-day class called "Fight Strong". A couple weeks before the class, James called to tell me about it and said, "You need to get your ass up here for this class, and bring Jarrad."

Having known James for better than ten years and respecting his opinions, I said "Okay, we'll be there." I had no idea that what I would learn that weekend would not only change my life, but potentially save it.

Matt Reynolds owns a company called Barbell Logic Online Coaching. He also conducts numerous seminars every year to teach people the scientifically proven, most efficient way to lift a barbell and gain physical strength, regardless of sex or age or physical condition. The method that Matt teaches has been proven to be effective for men and women, from teenagers to seniors in their seventies.

For two days in Tennessee, Matt focused on only four barbell lifts; the squat, bench press, overhead press (standing), and deadlift. He explained in detail the importance of form, body positioning, and all the seemingly minor details that go into lifting a barbell.

If you know anything about me, you know that I was a United States Marine. Needless to say, I have done my share of physical exercise and I have been in shape. I played a little football in high school and I practiced the martial arts, but I never really knew how I should lift a barbell and the specifics of that movement. I suppose, like many men, I just watched other people do it for years and tried to mimic what I saw.

This was different. I now understood the importance of all the little details and the importance of having a strength training coach to assist me. When I returned home to Biloxi, I began a genuine strength training program and documented every session.

When we moved from Mississippi to Wyoming it took a few weeks to get settled and set up a home gym at the new house, but I did it and I continued to make progress. On my one year anniversary of the Fight Strong class I referred back to my notes and was able to see the very real strength gains that I had made. This was not just a feel good program. At the time I was 50 years old and I was able to say, with all honesty, that I was lifting heavier weight than at any other time in my life.

Matt and his coaches were always there with support and encouragement. They critiqued my lifts via video and helped me to make the little changes I would have never realized on my own that I needed to make.

The day I got the cancer phone call was a work out day. Rather than throw a pity party for myself, I went downstairs to the gym and lifted the weight. When I got under that bar I knew I was not just lifting to meet a personal strength goal; I was lifting to save my life. That is how I continued to approach workout days. I was not going to give in to cancer. My plan was simply to force my body to rebuild and repair and be stronger every day until I could not do it anymore.

I kept up with my weight training routine as best I could. There were some overnight trips to the hospital and then the move to Utah, but nonetheless, I was able to keep lifting and getting stronger up until the point of being hospitalized. Though I don't want to come off as bragging, I was able to hit a PR (personal record) overhead press two weeks into my radiation treatments. From a psychological standpoint, that truly meant a lot to me and I felt that I was doing my part to fight el Cancer. (gratuitous Deadpool reference)

It is that type of purposeful and deliberate fighting, against gravity, to which I attribute much of the reason that I am still here and writing this book about my story.

When I started using the term "Fighting Solves Everything" I wasn't being glib or trying to be funny. Fighting Solves Everything is a definitive way of looking at the world and dealing with the troubles and adversities that come into every life.

In this particular situation I was dealing with the disease of cancer, but Fighting Solves Everything is not just about dealing with cancer. It just happens to work in that regard.

When people are diagnosed with cancer, the word fight gets thrown around all the time. "We are going to fight this." say the doctors and nurses. "Keep fighting, don't give up." say our friends and relatives. Everyone loves to use the word "fight" but what does that really mean?

If you simply surrender to the medical experts and wait for them to treat the cancer as they have decided, you are not really fighting. Laying on a table while Gamma radiation shoots through your body doesn't feel like fighting. Sitting for hours and hours in a chair while chemotherapy poison drips into your veins doesn't feel like fighting.

Everyone says fight, but no one ever tells you how to fight. Do you know what feels like fighting? Getting under a barbell and pushing back against the forces of gravity feels like fighting. Forcing yourself to push the weight, even though you are tired and depressed and would rather just go lay down; *that* is fighting. Looking at your notebook and realizing that despite having a deadly disease inside of your body, you lifted more weight today than you did last week. *That* feels like fighting. That is an accomplishment you cannot fake and something that no one can give you. You cannot purchase strength, no matter how much money you spend. Only you can win the fight against gravity.

The Treatment

Between April 15th, 2019 and the first week of May 2019, I had numerous appointments and consultations. The first one was with Dr Ying Hitchcock, Radiation Specialist. Then I was sent to Dr. Canon, Surgical Specialist, to determine whether or not surgery might be the answer to getting rid of the cancer.

Dr. Canon ran a scope down my right nostril to the back of my throat to get a close look at the tumor. It was determined that the primary disease was located on the farthest back portion of my tongue, but it was also affecting my lymph nodes and salivary glands on the right side of my neck. The tumor was "slightly past midline" on my tongue which meant that Dr. Canon would not recommend surgery. The amount of damage to the back of my throat, particularly my vocal chords, was not worth the risk. Surgery would also require removing the lymph nodes on both sides of my neck; something that would create a whole new set of problems. On a Friday morning in mid-April, the "Tumor Board" met, discussed my case, and decided to recommend a full battery of direct radiation oncology and chemotherapy.

This was the first time since being diagnosed that anyone had mentioned chemo. The doctors in Wyoming had said radiation, but never chemo. Now I needed to go in for a consultation with Dr. Weiss, the Chemotherapy Specialist. Dr. Weiss, explained that chemotherapy would not cure my type of cancer. I remember him saying, "I could give you chemo for a year and it would not kill the tumor." But, they felt that chemo, combined with radiation, would give me a 5-10 percent better chance of beating the disease.

Then came the battery of side effects. All the commonly understood side effects came first, nausea and vomiting, loss of appetite, loss of energy, dramatic weight loss, potential hair loss, neuropathy (pain, numbness, and weakness in fingers and toes) potential vision loss and hearing loss. Oh, don't forget severe kidney damage.

Consult number two that same day was the pharmacist who came in to explain the battery of anti-nausea medications that would be required to keep me from puking every day and generally feeling terrible.

I almost forgot, Dr. Chemo said that I would definitely need to have a feeding tube put in my stomach. We would have to schedule that simple surgery before treatment was started. Dr. Hltchcock had mentioned that some patients would get feeding tubes and some did not. I had told her that I would not. Dr. Chemo seemed very insistent that I get the tube procedure before we could start any treatment.

I left the hospital that day feeling genuinely depressed and more frustrated and angry than I had been up to this point. Right up to the time I talked to Dr. Chemo, all the doctors had said that the type of cancer I had was "highly treatable". Daily radiation treatments would take about 15 minutes for each session and then I could just go on with my day. The pain that would develop in my neck was described as a "bad sunburn".

My official cancer diagnosis had come on February 22, 2019. Here I was in the third week of April 2019 and not one step closer to treating the disease, save what I had been doing myself, the Keto diet and weight training.

It took only a few minutes to insert the type of chemo drug they wanted to give me into a search engine. What I discovered was a plethora of information about cisplatin. The instances of permanent hearing loss were listed as "40 to 80 percent of all patients experienced permanent hearing loss". Dr. Chemo seemed perfectly fine to have a living, deaf cancer survivor. "Wouldn't you rather be alive and deaf?" he asked.

I was also able to find medical papers and studies that suggested that adding chemotherapy to radiation as a treatment for my type of cancer was very likely "over-treatment", however, the medical community was waiting for more information before making that decision. My gut feelings combined with what I discovered about the side effects of cisplatin were enough for me to make the call, I would NOT be taking chemotherapy.

Nancy and I discussed my feelings and she agreed with me. She said she did not like what Dr. Chemo said and if I did not want to take chemo, she supported me. I took a deep breath and called Dr. Hitchcock's office. Rebecca, Dr. Hitchcock's primary nurse, took my phone call. I told Rebecca about my feelings and misgivings about chemotherapy and that I had decided I was not going to do it.

Rebecca would turn out to be a great help to us and a genuinely sympathetic ear. She said she understood my concerns and asked if I could hold on for just a moment, Dr. Hitchcock had just walked in. When she came back on the line a few minutes later she said she had expressed my concerns and that Dr. Hitchcock was totally fine with me not taking chemo.

This was a huge psychological relief. I had expected some push back and was prepared to go to war to defend my decision. It felt good to have someone in my corner at the hospital regarding this concern. Rebecca reconfirmed my next appointment. I would be going in for what they called a "dry run" on Monday May 6, 2019. For the dry run, I would meet my radiation team, they would take me through the procedure and be sure we were set to begin six weeks of radiation treatments, everyday, Monday through Friday.

Between my surgery consult and my chemotherapy consult, I had gone to the radiation area where I was fitted with my mask, my mouth guards, my head pillow, and given my three tattoo dots. For direct radiation oncology, or the "Gamma Knife" as they call it, the patient needs to be positioned in the machine within one millimeter of the same position every single time. As my cancer was in my neck/throat, my head would need to be immobilized so that it would always be in the same position when I climbed onto the machine each of the 30 different times I would do so.

A foam block was fitted to the back of my head. That would go onto the table first to keep my head steady. Then a polymer mesh mask was warmed up and stretched over my face and clamped to the table. In order to assure that my jaw bones were always in the same position, a double mouthguard, top and bottom, was conformed to my teeth. Lastly, the technician used black India ink and a needle to make three, small dot tattoos on me; one on each shoulder and one in the dead center of my upper chest. Everytime I would climb onto the radiation table I would bare my upper chest and the team would align the tattoo dots with three red lasers from the machine. My head would be in the foam cradle and they would hand me my mouthguard. Then the mask would be lowered over my face and secured to the table so I could not move at all. On the backboard were right and left peg handles for me to hold on to during the treatment.

True to their word, each radiation procedure took only about 15 minutes from the time I was secured to the table until they came back into the radiation room and released me. About halfway through the 30 treatments, Nancy came back in the room with me and watched them set me up on the machine as they explained the radiation procedure to her. One time was all she needed. She said she did not want to see it anymore.

Massive doses of radiation are obviously dangerous to the human body, which is why the Gamma Knife treatments are so short. However, the effects of the radiation are cumulative and they build up over time.

During the first week, I really did not notice much of a change. You do not feel anything during the treatment itself, not heat or pain. The only thing you hear is the machine moving and changing position. I kept my eyes closed during every treatment. The mesh mask impaired my view anyway and I didn't want to watch the machine which was only inches from my face.

One of the nice aspects of the treatment was the music selection. Thanks to Internet music players, a patient could pick out any type of music they wanted and have it piped into the speakers in the treatment room. In order to protect the staff from radiation exposure, no one is actually in the room with the patient. They monitor it all with cameras and video monitors, remotely, from outside the insulated room.

Each day when I showed up Dan, the head radiation tech, or one of his staff would ask me what kind of music I wanted to hear. I tried to mix it up a bit depending on my mood. Sometimes I would just ask them to put on 80's Rock and other times I would ask for a specific band. I was able to introduce my radiation team not only to Pop Evil, but to Kitaro as well. I was the teacher and we had music appreciation class each day when I arrived.

By the end of week two things in my mouth and throat had begun to change. My tastebuds were being damaged and day by day food started tasting bland. By week three, most food tasted like chalk or cardboard, or perhaps Play Doh. Oh, and as an added bonus, the smell of cooking food made me nauseous. It got so bad that I could not be anywhere near the kitchen when Nancy was cooking for the family because is made me horribly sick to my stomach.

Also, it was about this time that Nancy started noticing the radiation burns on my chest, neck, and my back below my head. And, that is about the time when the throat pain truly began.

By week three, swallowing was becoming difficult and painful, particularly when I tried to eat and chew up food. Liquids went down alright, but chewing and swallowing food was more difficult each day. My salivary glands were being damaged and not producing the saliva and enzymes needed to break down solid food. For pain we switched back and forth between Tylenol and Advil. We'd been advised not to use aspirin.

Also, during week three leading into week four, I truly started to lose my energy. Afternoon naps became mandatory in order to get through the day and my voice began to suffer. Most days I could only talk for a short time before it hurt too much to continue.

On Monday of week four my throat hurt so badly that over the counter pain medicine could not touch the pain. The pain was constant and kept me from sleeping. Nancy called the hospital and drove me to Huntsman early so I could see the doctor before my radiation treatment. I knew I could not lay perfectly still with a mouthguard in unless I had something for the pain.

One of the on-call doctors came in and sprayed my throat with some type of narcotic pain medicine. That knocked the pain back and I was able to get through my treatment. I did have to write my music selection down on a piece of paper as talking was difficult.

After the treatment we saw Dr. Hitchcock. She scolded me for waiting until Monday to come in and suffering all weekend. She said that if the pain ever became unbearable to go the the Huntsman ER. We left that day with a narcotic pain medicine prescription and instructions. During week four, however, my condition got worse and worse.

By the Friday of week four of radiation treatment, even the pain medicine they had given me was not working very well. My neck hurt to the point that it was extremely painful to even drink water. This was not a bad sunburn, it was pain like I had never experienced in my life.

The Study

During the initial consultation phase at Huntsman, before treatment began, Dr. Hitchcock asked me if I would be willing to participate in a cancer research study that Huntsman was conducting for people with my type of the disease. She explained that it would involve an MRI scan of me before any treatment began and then another one mid-way through.

Nancy and I discussed it and decided that as long as they didn't want to do something crazy, I might as well participate. We told Rebecca that I was in and she set up a phone call with the research people. It was not long before I received a phone call from a nice lady at the Radiation Testing and Lab facility. She explained that my participation would require a full MRI with an injected contrast conducted twice; once the week before my treatment began and then again approximately two to three weeks into my direct radiation oncology.

The woman also stated that there would be no cost to me or my insurance company (ha!) and that they would compensate me for my time. She was authorized to offer $50 per session for a total of $100. Woo Hoo! Better than a poke in the eye with a sharp stick. The main purpose of the phone call was to set an appointment for the first test, which we did.

When the day for my test MRI arrived, Nancy and I showed up about twenty minutes before the appointment time. They, of course, had asked me to get there early so I could fill out the obligatory paperwork. The nice lady from the phone handed me a clipboard. Because the test involved an MRI, the questionnaire form naturally had questions as to whether or not I had previously had surgeries where metal pins or screws were implanted in my body. They asked if I had any piercings or tattoos and where they were located on my body. One question asked if I had a "penile implant". Yes, the 13 year old in me thought that was funny. I drew a smiley face next to the question on the form and snapped a picture with my phone to share.

After completing the paperwork, I handed the nice lady the clipboard and she showed me to the changing room to put on the metal-free hospital clothing and special traction socks. When I came out of the changing room ten minutes later Nancy was sitting there with a half smirk, half scowl on her face. "What?" I said responding to her look. "You are such a child", she scolded me, but could not stop herself from laughing. It seemed that the nice lady needed some clarification about the penile implant question so she asked Nancy about it.

"What did you tell her?" I asked. "I said you were a child and no, you do not have one." If nothing else, I like to keep Nancy's life interesting.

The nice lady then escorted me to the testing area. First a technician came up and drew my blood to check my kidneys and then they put in an IV line for the contrast. I had been through a couple of MRI screenings about twenty years before. It is probably good that so much time had passed. If you have never been claustrophobic in your life, the MRI will bring that out of you.

Before being put in the machine I was introduced to the Radiology doctor in charge. I cannot remember her name, but she was obviously from somewhere in southeast Asia. I had to pay close attention to her to get everything she was saying. She thanked me for volunteering for the study.

Now it was time for the machine. The saving grace was the earbuds that the MRI techs put on me so I could try to listen to music over the deafening sounds of the machine. They also put a cradle over your head with an angled mirror so you can look out of the machine toward your feet. Otherwise it would feel like you were shoved into a noisy drain pipe.

As the backboard/table portion of the machine slid me inside, I closed my eyes and said the Lord's

Prayer. I also asked God to bless me and keep me from coughing or sneezing while inside the machine. Any movement or disturbance forces the tech to rescan and makes the test even longer.

I asked them to put on an 80's Rock station, which they did. The sound of the familiar music was comforting. I tried to focus on the music and not the anxiety of being trapped in a tube. I could hear the music until the machine kicked on and made all of the noise it makes. Oh, and just so you know, the MRI does not just make one type of noise that might allow you to get used to it. No, as soon as you get used to one type of noise, the machine changes up and starts with another disturbing sound. I imagine the CIA must use something similar to torture information out of spies and terrorists.

To be truthful, I had no idea how much time had passed when they pulled me out. I was just grateful to be finished. I was a bit groggy as I had drifted in and out of a sleep state. As always, Nancy was waiting for me out front. She informed me that I had been in the back for over an hour. The second MRI appointment was scheduled so that I would be just over two weeks into my radiation therapy. As a sign of the favor of God, I found a $20 bill lying on the ground behind our truck when we came out. No one was around but us.

The second MRI visit was nearly identical to the first, with the exception that I knew where everything was and Nancy filled out the paperwork. Once more, I was given contrast and put in the machine with earbuds and music playing. Yes, again, I said the Lord's Prayer and asked God to calm my soul. By this time I was becoming quite the practiced patient.

As I would learn when I was finished in the claustrophobia machine, the nice lady sat down with Nancy in the waiting room and inquired as to how she was doing, how she was holding up. Also, the Radiology doctor came out to talk with Nancy. She thanked Nancy for bringing me in and told her that there were not that many people participating in the study. More importantly, the doctor had been in the MRI booth observing as they scanned me. She saw the size of the tumor three weeks earlier and she remarked to Nancy that the tumor was noticeably smaller during my second MRI than it had been during the first.

That news was great to hear. I felt reassured that the treatments were working and we were on the right path. I might also add that up to that point, no one on my team at Huntsman had mentioned anything of the sort. I suppose in their minds the treatment was just going to work, so no point in talking about it.

Hospitalized

Most people who receive cancer treatment do so on an outpatient plan. Staying overnight in the hospital is not a normal part of the treatment procedure. On Saturday morning of week four of my treatment I was in bad shape. The pain had kept me awake most of the night. I was not able to drink anything, much less eat. I knew that I could not wait until Monday because I would dehydrate and get even sicker.

Nancy called the Huntsman Emergency Room number, explained that I was a cancer patient undergoing treatment and explained what was going on. The advice was simple; get him here as soon as you can.

My beloved bride loaded me into our pickup truck to drive me the short distance to the ER. I had a red Solo cup with a paper towel stuffed in it. My throat was so inflamed that it hurt to swallow my own saliva.

We arrived at the Huntsman ER shortly after 9 a.m. and they were able to get me back in the exam room pretty quickly. We might have sat in the lobby for fifteen or twenty minutes. After a nurse took my vitals, the first doctor came in and had a look at my throat. "It's definitely infected." he said. I asked if that would cause additional pain, more so than the radiation treatments? "Oh, yes most definitely." Great! (heavy sarcasm implied)

They moved me back to a treatment room and started an IV. It was apparent that I was beginning to get dehydrated. They also gave me a shot of some strong narcotic medicine to knock back the throat pain. Once I was stabilized they had time to consult with the doctors at the Cancer Center about what to do with me. It being Saturday, Dr. Hitchcock was off duty and an on-call doctor for the Radiation department would be fielding my case.

Nancy waited with me in the Emergency Department treatment room for hours. I kept trying to convince her to go and get something to eat as I knew she had to be hungry, or at least a cup of coffee. She only accepted water from the nurse. They dimmed the lights in the room and I fell asleep.

After a few hours in the treatment room, a new doctor came in to tell me that they had consulted with the Cancer Center doctors and they felt it would be best to keep me, at least for one night, to try and get the infection under control and to get enough fluids in me to be safe.

Not very long after that an attendant showed up with a wheelchair. The Huntsman Cancer Center and Hospital occupies a lot of real estate. The

Emergency Department was down the hill a bit from the Cancer Center, several hundred yards at least. What I learned was that most of the buildings were interconnected by covered walkways. After about fifteen minutes, maybe longer, I was wheeled onto the 5th floor of the Huntsman Cancer Center where the overnight hospital rooms were located.

I have not been in a lot of hospital rooms in my life. Before el Cancer, it had been eighteen years since I spent a night in a hospital. My room at Huntsman was extremely nice. All the cabinets and furniture were hardwood or looked like hardwood. There was a long couch built in to the far wall below a bay window that took up the entire outside wall. Huntsman sits high up in the hills on the eastern side of Salt Lake City. My view from the room was the western mountains and the city in the valley below. I did not want to be in the hospital, but if I had to be in one, this was a good one to be in.

Nancy moved the truck from the ER parking lot up the hill to the Cancer Center lot and met me in my 5th floor room. Only one other time during my seven days in the hospital would she leave and go out of the building.

By the time I was settled in my room, it was late on Saturday afternoon. The primary mission of the nurses was to keep my pain under control, get fluid into my body via IV and monitor my blood pressure and respiration. This proved a chore. The narcotic pain medicine worked so well that I would fall asleep deeply and my breathing would drop so low that it would set off the monitor alarm. Of course, the alarm would snap me out of my sleep and I would breathe deeply, but that didn't help me rest.

In the morning, the attending doctor came in to see me. He confirmed that I had a serious infection in my throat, combined with the radiation damage, this was causing me the tremendous pain. The doctor assured me that the infection was a common side effect of the radiation treatment (Yea!) and it was easily treated with an antibiotic liquid.

I had not eaten anything since Friday, and that was a protein shake. By Monday morning the doctors had decided that I would need a feeding tube. The options were twofold; a nose tube or a stomach tube. The nose tube was less invasive as it did not require surgery, but there would be a tube sticking out of my left nostril taped to the side of my head; super attractive. The stomach tube would be installed via a simple surgical procedure, but it did entail cutting a hole in my abdomen and stomach to insert the tube.

This is where the hospital doctors and Dr. Hitchcock collided. Hitchcock said nose tube, hospital doctors said stomach tube. For my part, I was weak and starving and unsure what would be best. They decided to try the nose tube and I consented.

The nose tube technician came to my room sometime in the early afternoon. She sprayed some numbing agent in my left nostril and then proceeded to snake a tube down my nasal passage (I swallowed hard) then into my esophagus and down to my stomach. The entire procedure took about fifteen minutes. It felt weird having a tube sticking out of my face, but at the time I was just rolling with. The plan was to leave the tube alone for a few hours and let me get used to it, then have the 2nd shift nurse try and feed me through the tube.

A lot of my time in the hospital blended together. After the first couple of days it all seemed the same. However, I remember the evening they tried to feed me through the nose tube. The 2nd shift nurse came in around 7 p.m. I think. She had a carton of something, probably an Ensure type liquid meal, and she hooked up a small funnel to the end of my nose tube. The plan was simple; hold the end of the tube upright, slowly pour the liquid in, let gravity take it to my stomach. Nancy, as always, was there with me.

The nurse began to slowly pour some water in the hose. When it reached my stomach I immediately felt nauseous. I asked her if it should be making me sick. She said no, but the feeling would probably pass. She added a little bit more and that is when my body said 'No'.

With little to no warning, I was seized by a vomiting attack. Everything in my stomach, the liquid, some blood, and the tube came violently out of my mouth. I vomited the nose tube out of my mouth and that caused a choking/gagging reaction. Instinctively, I tried to get the object that was choking me out of my mouth. However, the tube was secured to the outside of my face with a tie that went through my nose. Fortunately, the nurse had a pair of medical shears in her pocket. She reached up and cut the tube at my mouth and pulled the remainder out of my nose and my throat.

I felt terrible that I had made just a horrible mess. My hospital gown and the bed sheets were covered in vomit and blood. I know this is more than for which you, the readers, bargained. Sorry. I hated that Nancy had to see that go down. She was right there with me and put her arm around me to comfort me.

It was not just Nancy for whom I felt bad. I felt bad for the nurse who had tried to feed me and then had to cut the nose tube out of me to keep me from ripping it out. All of the nurses and aids were very nice and professional. Like you will find with all people, some expressed more concern than others.

The nurses rotated not only shifts but room responsibilities so there were several different people, maybe ten to twelve who attended to me in the hospital. A couple of the nurses, even though I was not on their rotation, popped in during the week to check on me. That was genuinely kind.

There was another genuine act of kindness that I want to relate. During my radiation treatments, a couple members of my team changed. Huntsman is a teaching hospital, so change in personnel is not surprising. During week 5 of radiation, which was the week of my hospital stay, I was strapped to the Gamma Knife table and my procedure had just begun when the lights flickered. It was a momentary power outage.

Dan came into the treatment room and confirmed the power outage and let me know that the machines, and the computers that operated them, would all need to be reset. Would I mind holding on and staying in position? I made a "yes" sound through my double mouthguard. My head was immobilized as per usual so I could not get up even if I wanted to. Dan left me alone in the quiet room.

After a few moments, a young lady, I'm a total jerk because I cannot remember her name, came in. She had just started with my radiation team the day before. She let me know that they expected it to take ten to fifteen more minutes before the machines were ready to go. I had been strapped to the table for much longer than normal by this time. Sympathetic to my plight, she asked if I would like her to stay with me until the machines were back up.

Once more, through my mouthguard, I mumbled "yes". She stood next to me and took my right hand in hers. It was a simple and kind gesture, a warm expression of caring that she was certainly not required to do, but she did nonetheless. That expression of kindness warms my heart every time I think about it.

Back to the feeding tube story. Lesson learned. The nose tube was not going to work. A stomach tube would be the answer. They just needed to get me on the surgery schedule as soon as possible. I had not eaten for four days and I was losing weight now more than ever.

I was still undergoing radiation treatment while I was in the hospital, but the commute was much shorter. Each morning about fifteen minutes before my scheduled radiation treatment a young man or woman would arrive with a wheelchair and cart me down to the first floor for my treatment. Then they would come back when I was done and take me back to my room.

In the afternoons and evenings, Nancy and I would take a stroll around the 5th floor. We would make a couple of laps. The majority of the time I was hooked up to an IV pole, so we had to push that around. It was better than lying in bed 24 hours a day. The 5th floor had a designated Lactation Room. I kept trying to get Nancy to take me in there, but she wouldn't go for it.

Once again, if my memory serves me, it was Wednesday afternoon when they were able to get me on the surgery schedule for my stomach tube insertion. This time they just wheeled me down in my bed. The bed was pulled up right next to the operating table so they could easily shift me over. The entire procedure seemed like something from a dream. I had been given pain medicine right before. They did not knock me out but I remember having oxygen put on my face. I drifted in and out for a while and the next thing I knew they were telling me that I was going back to my bed and that we were all done. Nancy was there waiting for me when I came back to the room with my new friend; Mr. Feeding Tube.

After the stomach tube was in place, the rest of my time in hospital was like Groundhog Day. Each day the doctors would come in and check on my condition. The primary concern was to be sure the feeding tube was working without complications and that I was hydrated and moving my bowels.

They also adjusted my pain and nausea medicine several times.

Nancy still laughs when she tells this story, but during the first couple of days they gave me medicine for nausea that literally caused me to have hallucinations. I would slip back and forth between a dream state and consciousness. More than once I thought I saw strangers standing in the room with us. During one episode, I asked Nancy about the pilot who had been in the room with us and said something to the effect of having flown to the hospital on an airplane.

As comical as this was, Nancy told the staff that they needed to stop giving me that medicine because it was "making me crazy". By the time I would leave the hospital the following Saturday they had figured out which nausea medicine would not cause hallucinations and they had me on a new pain medicine regime. This would include a 50 mcg Fentanyl patch and Dilaudid tablets to bridge the gap. Yes, by the time I would be discharged, my body would be physically addicted to narcotic pain medicine. But that was just how it had to be.

The good news was that radiation treatment week 5 was completed before I left the hospital. I had started my 30 treatments on a Tuesday and there was one holiday break in between. When I got back home I only had 7 radiation appointments left. There was light at the end of the tunnel.

Nutrition

As I mentioned in an earlier chapter, prior to commencing treatment we had a number of different referrals and consultations. During one visit, I met with a "Speech and Swallow" therapist. She was a super nice lady who gave me swallowing exercises to practice as the ability to swallow would be more and more difficult as time went by.

After the Speech Therapist visit we had a consultation with the "Dietary Specialist". During our initial interview Nancy explained that I was on the Keto diet and had been since my first diagnosis. To that the Dietician scoffed and essentially said that it was a fad diet and I didn't need to be losing weight. She also stated that the body would naturally convert fat and protein to carbohydrates for energy, so depriving the body of sugar and carbs was pointless. Yep, she said that.

Then she followed up the previous statement by saying that their prime concern was me losing muscle mass, as that was common in cancer patients going through treatment. Her suggestion to help me maintain muscle mass? Eat lots of potatoes, peanut butter, and try tofu. Yes, she said tofu; soybean curd. When I said "No thanks, I don't think I need artificial estrogen in my diet." She responded that it was a "myth" that soy had estrogen properties.

There you have it. The professional dietician suggested that I consume soy, peanut butter, and potatoes to help maintain my muscle mass. Oh, I almost forgot. She also gave us a handout that suggested we avoid red meat due to the risk of heart disease from eating it. Nancy and I left that appointment considerably disappointed and annoyed.

To her great credit, when I had to get on Keto, Nancy did a tremendous amount of research. It seemed painfully obvious that this "Dietary Specialist" was reading from a woefully outdated playbook. It is not red meat that causes heart disease, but a constant corn diet and inflammation that causes fat to build up around the heart.

We told the dietician that I was engaging in serious strength training, you know, to build and maintain muscle mass, and she seemed unphased and did not even know what to do with that information. *You mean you are lifting heavy barbells to force your body to rebuild and grow muscle? Why would you do that? Just increase your peanut butter and tofu intake.*

Perhaps five or six weeks after the first dietician appointment, we encountered another Nutrition

Specialist while I was in the hospital. This woman had an office on the 5th floor and I would not meet her until my feeding tube was installed.

She came in on the first day of my tube placement to talk with Nancy and I about what to feed me through the tube. The first thing she suggested were the premade cans of "Boost" and "Ensure". If you take the time to read the ingredients in these products, not only are they not Keto-friendly, they are packed with filler crap. Soy protein is the key ingredient. They also have sucralose, yes, going back to the Keto chapter, artificial sweeteners are akin to "miracle grow" for tumors. What the Actual Fuck? A Nutrition Specialist in a Cancer Treatment hospital suggests that cancer patients be fed a diet of soy protein and artificial sweetener, three to four times a day.

A disgusting fact that I learned from being around other cancer patients, many of whom had stomach feeding tubes, was that many of these poor souls had horrible, foul smelling diarrhea. Why you might be wondering? Chemotherapy? Yes. And, as I would learn from the nurses who treated them, a steady tube feed diet of Ensure and Boost made their BM's loose and foul. Wonderful!

Nancy, being as patient as she could be, explained to Nutrition Lady that I was eating Keto AND that, in my case, I could not eat soy anything. I have not mentioned it yet, but my body has had a soy (and any lentils/beans) intolerance since I was a young child. Soy anything, baked beans, peanuts, etc. make me extremely sick. So, no I would not be taking liquid soy protein through my feeding tube.

This fact stumped Nutrition Lady, who apparently had the same outdated playbook as the other Dietician. What could we do? Well, we could talk to the ladies in the kitchen and see if they could come up with a blended tube food minus soy, etc. What the kitchen came up with was a blend of instant mashed potatoes, peaches, and a few other ingredients.

Nutrition Lady also told Nancy that we would need large 2 ounce syringes to feed the food into my stomach tube. We could buy them directly from the hospital for $5 a piece. Yes, you read that right, it was not a typo, $5 each for disposable plastic syringes. Nancy found them on Amazon for 50 cents a piece and we bought in bulk. We went through dozens and dozens.

For the last few days in the hospital, we made due with the tube food that the kitchen produced for us. Before we even left, Nancy started researching and coming up with tube food recipes to ensure that I would be getting fat, protein, oils, vitamins, and a small amount of carbohydrates in my tube. I was able to eat one small Jello cup in the hospital, that was all I ate by mouth for a week.

One of the primary reasons for this book to exist is the addition of the recipe section at the end. Nancy learned a tremendous amount, not only about the Keto diet, but about how to get me good, nutritious food through a feeding tube. None of that information came from the professionals at the Cancer Treatment center. We had to go about it the hard way and learn by trial and error. The Keto diet does not have to be as difficult as people think it is and Nancy has numerous recipes to help you out.

Faith

As discussed earlier in this book, I have a strong faith in God and have had my entire life. This is primarily due to the upbringing my parents provided and the church family that was a large part of my formative years.

Regardless of how strong your faith might be, the grim reality of mortality, particularly when it is thrust in your face as cancer does, can shake anyone's faith. I had many prayerful conversations with the Almighty. Primarily, I asked for the strength to do what needed to be done and to see me through to whatever outcome might be in front of me.

Some of the most difficult times, at least emotionally, were the few weeks of uncertainty before we had a treatment plan in place, the "you have cancer, but we are not sure how bad or where it is" time. From a physical standpoint, I felt good. I felt healthy. But emotionally, there was a huge weight on my shoulders.

Nancy prayed with me and for me unceasingly. As I mentioned earlier, I told very few people of the diagnosis until I had a treatment plan. I could not see the point in a phone call that went; "Hi, I have cancer. No, I don't have a treatment plan yet. Just thought you would want to know so you could be worried and feel like shit." That was not how I wanted my parents and family to know about my cancer.

After the initial shock of the diagnosis wore off, I felt like God was directing my way toward treatment. Being in Saratoga, Wyoming complicated the treatment plan. We were going to have to move, that was a given. I truly believe it was the favor of God that Jarrad had just moved into a house that had extra bedrooms and was only a fifteen minute drive away from the cancer treatment center. I would learn later that many patients at Huntsman Cancer Center commuted from great distances to get treatment. As bad as I felt during the latter weeks of radiation treatment, having to sit in a car for an hour or more would have made it worse.

We had to close the Saratoga office of Student of the Gun, obviously. Again, we had the favor of God that Jarrad was working in an office in the Readyman / Black Rifle Coffee building. My good friend, Jeff Kirkham, mentioned before, made sure that we had the space we needed to work 100 percent out of SLC and that included our shipping department.

Once a treatment plan was in place, I made the cancer diagnosis public. I knew I would have to take time off from the radio and production and that it would be noticed. Rather than just mysteriously disappear for a month or two, I thought it would be better to be honest and upfront with the audience.

To this day I am humbled and touched emotionally to the point of tears at the outpouring of love and support and prayers that I received from hundreds and thousands of people whom I have never met. After I was given the all clear from the doctors, I remarked that with the thousands of people praying on my behalf, that cancer did not have a chance. Christ our savior said, "where two or three gather in my name, I am there with them." Matthew 18:20. He was certainly there with me in the waiting rooms of so many doctors offices and hospitals, on the table under the radiation machine, inside of the MRI and PET Scan machines, when I was laid up in a hospital bed, and all during my recovery.

When the radiation treatment began, I set my mind on the fact that it would succeed and that the tumor would be killed. While there might have been a bit of nagging worry in the back of my mind as the final scan approached, I did not dwell on the possibility that the treatment would not work.

The decision to deny the chemotherapy came after much prayer on both mine and Nancy's part. I told Rebecca, Dr. Hitchcock's nurse, that I was not afraid to die and I genuinely meant it. I was not being glib. I know that He has a mansion waiting for me as He promised. Again, I understand that for many cancer patients, chemotherapy is the number one treatment. For me, I knew that it was not.

One of our close followers sent a little wooden cross. The cross was something he kept with himself during his own cancer fight and he passed it on to me for mine. Now, being cancer free, I wear a sterling silver cross around my neck as a constant reminder of God's never ending grace, courtesy of that same man. The little wooden cross has been passed on to another man who is dealing with el Cancer now, and I hope it gives him the comfort it gave me.

A habit that I have tried to maintain and that I was sure to keep up all during those long days of treatment was to read my Bible daily. One Proverb a day was a minimum. Remember, there are 31 chapters in the book of Proverbs, one for each day of the month. I also read the New Testament as well as the Old.

While I was in the hospital, a man knocked on the door and asked if I had a moment to talk. He was a volunteer for the Hospital Chaplain and he asked if I might benefit from talking with the Chaplain. I told him that I would welcome a visit from the Chaplain and the next day he came to my room to visit. We talked for a bit and I shared my faith with him. He asked if I would like to take Holy Communion and I said that I did. My only regret was that people kept coming to the door and knocking during the private service. For as much as they tell you to rest in the hospital, there are always people knocking on the door.

But seek first his kingdom and his righteousness, and all these things will be given to you as well. Therefore do not worry about tomorrow, for tomorrow will worry about itself. Each day has enough trouble of its own. Matthew 6:33-34

Avoiding the Victim Mentality

When you are smacked with the news that you have a potentially deadly disease, it is quite natural to get down and feel sorry for yourself. Everyone experiences that initially, "Why me?" "It's not fair." Regardless, you need to find a way to get over that as quickly as you can and fight diligently against the victim mentality.

The one thing that I did not want to ever become was a "cancer patient". I know that sounds silly because, technically, from the moment I was given my diagnosis, I was on paper a cancer patient. I asked Nancy not to tell anyone and I instructed the kids to do the same thing. No social media posts, etc. about "Dad has cancer." I did not want people to treat me differently. I did not want the "Oh, poor guy, he's got cancer" looks of pity.

Yes, it was absolutely inevitable that it would get out that I was going through treatment. I tried the best I could to keep the victim mentality to an absolute minimum. One of the first ways I committed to not acting like a victim was to keep up my barbell training routine. There was no way I was going to let the diagnosis become a mental excuse not to train.

When discussing the Keto diet with Jeff and Dr. Dan, they both stated that it was common for people with cancer to start Keto and then quit as soon as it got hard or became inconvenient. They allow themselves to participate in a pity party or accept the role of victim. "If I'm going to have cancer, I'm going to eat whatever makes me happy."

It would have made me happy to eat pizza and pig out on ice cream or corn chips, but that was not going to help my body to heal itself. Maintaining a strict Keto diet was a part of my offensive fight against the cancer in my body and a way to avoid the victim mentality.

Another aspect of the fight was not to look like a cancer patient. Let's face reality. People sitting around in a waiting room wearing the typical ill-fitting hospital gowns look like sick people. I was going to have to sit in the waiting room, five days a week, for at least six weeks (turned out to be seven weeks because of holidays). I knew I did not want to look at myself in the mirror in one of those hospital gowns.

Fortunately for me, I have a wonderful wife and a fantastic mother. The first day I went for a scan at Huntsman Cancer Center I told Nancy that I hated the hospital gowns because they made me look like a cancer patient. My mother has been a skilled seamstress my entire life and she used to own and operate a medical uniform store. Nancy reached out to my mom and told her how I felt. A priority mail envelope arrived two days later with a men's navy blue scrub top (medical uniform). This one was for me to try on, to ensure fit and function.

For my radiation treatment I needed only to bare my upper chest. Therefore I would wear whatever pants I had on and a hospital gown, or in my case a scrub top, into the radiation treatment room.

Within a week, I received another priority package from my mother. This one had three new scrub tops. She used the manly material she had on hand to sew them together. The icing on the cake was a scrub top made from material with the United States Marine Corp Eagle, Globe and Anchor icon. I proudly wore my USMC scrub top to treatment the next day and received many compliments.

My first day in the hospital they put a generic gown on me, but Nancy soon retrieved my manly, non-victim shirts so that, even though I was sick as hell, I would not have to look the part of the cancer victim.

Many of you might think this is some kind of ego thing or a silly simplicity. I can assure you that for me it was not silly or small. Refusing to look the part of the cancer patient was another part of my fighting program. Apparently, I was one of the first patients to behave in such a way. Most every person I encountered on the Huntsman staff, when seeing my custom scrubs for the first time, commented about how much they liked them and asked me about the choice.

Just because you drew the short straw and were cursed with cancer does not mean you have to accept it and be cancer's bitch. From the very beginning I made the mental commitment that if anything was going to be a bitch, it was going to be that tumor in my neck. Refusing to look the part of the cancer patient was a statement that I chose to make. Also, for those of you who might be thinking "I'm not allowed to wear my own scrubs." or "The hospital staff won't approve." Number one, I never encountered any negative reaction to my choice, not one single time and number two, fuck anyone who would say something negative. Who the hell wants to wear a gown someone died in last week? Not me.

Another method that I employed to keep my mental spirits up and reduce the tendency to fall into the "victim mentality" was to listen to motivational music. Now, the music that motivates me may not be the music that motivates you and that is fine.

Each time I was scheduled for a radiation treatment I would first go to the men's changing room and put on my scrub top. They had individual lockers for your belongings. Each locker had keys on a curly plastic wristband. After changing, I would sit in a waiting room to await a member of my radiation team to come and fetch me.

There was a television that would have some inane garbage playing, such as CNN or some sports channel. If I entered the waiting room and I was alone, I would turn it off. About half the time there would be other patients in hospital gowns awaiting their turns. The radiation section has numerous treatment rooms, so it was possible to have multiple people getting treatment in the same time period that I was.

I made a habit of always having my earbuds and listening to some type of motivating music while I was waiting for my turn. This made the wait time go quickly and I did not sit there thinking about cancer and sickness and how crappy I might have felt at that time. The earbuds also saved me from having to listen to the inane drivel coming out of the idiot box on the wall.

Support Network

I have been extremely fortunate in my life to have several close friends. The kinds of friends that I might not talk with for a month or even a year but, at any given moment, pick right back up like we just saw each other yesterday.

When I finally made my diagnosis public, I was a bit overwhelmed and needed to send out text messages and emails to my friends telling them that "before you hear a rumor that I am sick, I am". For several days, I was on the phone constantly with friends letting them know what the plan for treatment and the outlook was.

James Yeager, of Tactical Response, was one of the first people to call me after I let the cat out of the bag on the Grad Program Bonus Hour. I should have told all of my friends first but, in my defense, this was my first time having cancer so I was learning as I was going along.

James asked me how I was feeling, what my insurance situation was like, and what my plans were for treatment. Like most small business owners, my insurance plan was "self-pay". Paying out of pocket for a private insurance plan was far too cost prohibitive to be practical; thank you Democrat Party and weak, spineless Republicans. The sick irony of the situation was that Nancy and I had insurance our entire married lives, right up until the year I got cancer. Yes, tens of thousands of dollars were paid to insurance companies to cover us and when we really needed it most, we did not have it.

In regards to the "self-pay" response, James asked if I had set up a "Go Fund Me" or something similar. I replied that I did not want to be "cancer boy" and ask people for money. At that moment James said I was being a rockhead, I was too close to the situation and he would work with Jarrad directly. I agreed to simply be the patient and focus on getting better. Jarrad and James would work on keeping me out of the poor house.

For the next several months, I received notes and actual physical cards from not just my friends, but from people I had never met. Many gifts arrived to help keep up my spirits and offer me encouragement. Like the prayers, I was overwhelmed again by the outpouring of support.

My friends would ask if there was anything they could do for me and the truth was that their expressions of support and encouragement were tremendously appreciated. I never felt alone or lonely. I knew that there were dozens of my friends in my corner. They checked in with me frequently by phone and then when I lost my voice via text.

The Recovery

As discussed during the previous chapter about The Treatment, the radiation made me nauseous, ruined my sense of taste, gave me radiation burns on the outside and on the inside causing tremendous pain, made my facial hair and some of the hair on my head fall out, and generally weakened my body.

After seven weeks and thirty individual radiation treatments I was moved into the "recovery phase". Based upon what I had been told, it would take "a couple of weeks" for me to start feeling better. During a follow up appointment the doctor said "a couple of months" before you start to feel normal. Yes, we went from a couple of weeks to a couple of months. Then, another doctor said, "expect to be dealing with symptoms for six months or more".

For the first couple of weeks post-radiation I felt weak and tired. I slept away most of the month of June and into July. The radiation caused my throat to produce excess mucus (I know, nasty) and I was constantly spitting it out. I had to keep a red plastic cup with paper towels stuffed in it, as a disposable spittoon, nearby at all times.

My energy level was drastically reduced. Nancy and I would go for walks around the block in our neighborhood. After about three-quarters of a mile I was worn out. Fortunately, I was able to sleep. During the first couple of months of recovery, I would sleep on average twelve hours a day.

Before I got very far into my treatment, I had planned to do a lot of reading and writing during my forced downtime. The reality that I discovered was that the pain medication I was on made it very difficult to focus mentally. I found that I could not focus on writing projects for more than about thirty minutes. As for reading, that was about the same, thirty minutes of reading was about all I could accomplish in one sitting.

It did not take very long for me to become frustrated. I wanted very badly to get back to work. I felt as though I was wasting my time and letting people down. To be honest, I could barely speak at all after my 30th radiation treatment and it was weeks before I could have a normal conversation without severe throat pain. To her great credit, Nancy started following online support groups for people who had the same cancer treatment as mine. Nancy assured me that, compared to other people in the same situation, I was recovering on pace, if not sooner than others.

Because I was on narcotic pain medicine, I had regularly scheduled check ups with the pain management team. During my first 30 day check up I erroneously thought they would be giving me the

"All Clear". To my chagrin, I was informed that, due to the amount of damage that the radiation had done to my throat, I would need to recover for 90 days before they would even attempt another scan to check for remaining cancer. That was a kick in the gut. I would have to wait another two months before I would know if the treatment had worked.

I had no reason to believe that the treatment did not work and I had faith that it did. It was just frustrating. Friends and family would constantly ask, "What did the doctors say?" in hopes that I could give them an all clear, cancer-free answer. Instead, I was stuck with the more complicated explanation.

My post-treatment PET Scan was set for September 11, 2019 in the morning. I know, quite an anniversary. Then I had a follow up appointment with the cancer doctor, Dr. Canon, in the afternoon that same day. I would see Dr. Hitchcock on Friday the 13th of September for my final consult with her.

During the recovery we started weaning me off of the opioid pain medication. When I left the hospital they had me on elephant strength pain meds to deal with the pain in my throat. For those in the know, or might know in the future, they had me on a 50 mcg Fentanyl patch with Dilaudid tablets to get me through the pain spikes.

The pain management doctor put me on a plan to reduce the patch by 25 percent each month. We dropped from 50 to 37 to 25 to finally a 12 mcg patch and then down to dilaudid 4 mg twice daily. Finally, we dropped to 2 mg twice daily, and then nothing.

It was not until I had been off the Fentanyl patch for a week that I realized that my throat was still causing me pain. It hurt in the exact area where the Gamma Knife had killed the tumor, but the pain meds had been covering it up. Now, minus any narcotics, the pain was back, though not as severe as it had been during treatment. We would work on numbing the pain by rotating Advil, Tylenol, and the numbing throat spray. However, none of the over the counter pain medicine could touch it.

Although it was again frustrating, I had to make a decision; be in constant pain or go back on the dilaudid pills. As bad as I wanted to be off the medicine, the throat pain was keeping me from sleeping and inhibiting my ability to work. Nancy and I talked and we realized I needed to give my throat more time to heal.

Not surprisingly, my body became quite physically addicted to the opioid pain medicine. Withdrawal symptoms from opioids are very real. For me, the withdrawal felt like the flu. I experienced severe aching in my large muscle groups, particularly in my legs, arms, and shoulders. I felt a genuine lethargy and lack of energy.

Opioid withdrawal sucks, but I wanted to get it all out of my system as soon as I could. When I stopped taking any and all opioid pain medicine my body was not happy. The muscle aches and pain were constant for several days. Unlike normal pain, where you can just lie still for relief, lying still, for me, did not help. The pain throbbed and kept me awake. Again, Nancy was my savior. She selflessly rubbed my aching legs and applied oils to them to help the muscles relax.

A big part of my mental and physical recovery was to get back into the gym and lift barbells as soon as I was able to do so. From the time I was hospitalized in early June to the middle of July I did not lift. When I went back to the gym to lift for the first time post-treatment I had lost exactly fifty pounds of body weight since receiving the diagnosis. Most of the weight came off after week three of radiation when my throat became inflamed and I ended up with a feeding tube.

July 15, 2019 was my first day back in the gym post-treatment. I still had the stomach tube in and I needed to be cautious about how much pressure I put on my abdomen. I parked my ego and started from the very beginning; I squatted an empty bar, bench pressed an empty bar, and put ten pound plates on the bar to deadlift. My goal was to try and perform the lifts as best as I could. I sent the videos to Graham and Matt, my coaches, and told them I was ready to get back into it. They both cautioned me to let them know if I experienced any sharp pain during the lifts. I agreed and began my second round of Linear Progression.

Because I had a stomach tube, I did not want to try and put a weight belt on or near it. My progression was slow but constant, adding five pounds to each exercise for each training session. Yes, there was a bit of mental frustration. I was frustrated to have lost so much progress from before el Cancer. My coaches cautioned me not to try and compare my current progress with my previous progress. I knew they were right, but it still irked me that fucking cancer had stolen so much of my strength.

As far as eating is concerned, I did not ever try to force food down my throat until July. Then we started with clear soup/broth, oatmeal, and other super soft and wet foods. I was able to drink clear liquids in early July and progressed to hot tea. My taste buds had been wiped out by the radiation, but mercifully they were coming back. I soon discovered that my taste buds were like those of a toddler. I could not tolerate spicy, salty, or bitter foods. I had stopped drinking coffee during week three of treatment and I now found the taste was too strong.

By August, I was able to chew and swallow soft foods like macaroni, yogurt, jello, pudding, etc. Nancy tried to blend up solid food into soupy concoctions, but the flavor was too much for me to tolerate. She did find protein shakes (Premier Protein), in various flavors, that were whey, not soy, and tasted good. By September first I was taking in at least half of my daily calories by mouth and the other half, plus medication, by tube.

The tube turned out to be a blessing and a curse. It was a blessing as it allowed me to get all of the nutrition and medication I needed. The curse part was the restrictions that came with it. I could not be far from home for very long. It wasn't like I could pull into a McDonalds and say "Can you blend up a cheeseburger and put it in a cup for me?"

For those that are wondering if I stayed Keto with the tube in my stomach, the answer is yes, for the most part. Everything that went into the tube was purposeful and deliberate; protein, fat, fiber, oils, vitamins, etc.

As I mentioned previously, Nancy was actively following the progress of other people who had the same kind of cancer treatment as I did. Many of them, at the same stage I was in, had not recovered their sense of taste or could eat any solid food. More than a few were still on pain medicine six months after completing their treatments. Nancy was encouraged at my progress and shared that with me.

In addition to what we have already discussed, I had an ace in the hole, so to speak. Dr. Dan not only advised me to get on the Keto diet immediately, but to get my testosterone level checked and potentially get testosterone therapy. While I was still in Saratoga, I had my annual "Man Physical" along with blood work. While I was in the office, I asked the doctor if she could have them check my testosterone levels as well.

When we arrived in Salt Lake City, I had the blood test and testosterone test results already completed. Dr. Dan suggested that I find a BioTe certified doctor. As you should understand, as men age, their testosterone levels drop, after age 40 they drop dramatically. It turned out that there were several BioTe doctors in the SLC area.

I made an appointment with a BioTe doctor, Monica Bell, and it was a simple process to have my Saratoga doctor fax the test results to her. Nancy and I went for a consult with Dr. Bell. After chatting for about a half hour about my options, I decided to get the treatment. There are several ways to get testosterone therapy, one of the newest is time release pellets. The number of pellets are based upon age, weight, and T level. Once inserted, they take about 30 days to fully kick in and last about six months. No creams or weekly shots.

I was in week two of radiation when I received my BioTe testosterone pellet treatment. We scheduled an appointment for 30 days after to check my levels. As it would turn out, the timing was good. By the time I finished my radiation treatments, I could use any help I could get for recovery. For the curious, yes, I was definitely able to realize when the testosterone started kicking in to my system.

The Results

During the three months between the end of radiation treatment and my PET Scan I was able to get back to work. At first I was only able to talk for an hour or two per day before my throat would get sore and my voice would give out.

We had scheduled a training course, Beyond the Band Aid, for the first weekend in September thinking that I would be fully healed by then. As the date for the course approached I was a bit nervous as I was still experiencing throat discomfort and had not talked that much for that long in months.

I prayed to God and asked him to bless my voice and give me the ability to deliver the material. Sixteen students had traveled from great distances to be here in Salt Lake City. Not surprisingly, my prayers were answered and I was able to talk well enough to get through two, eight hours days. Jeff Kirkham helped me out greatly by delivering the tourniquet lecture.

The Wednesday after that class was September 11, 2019. Nancy drove me to Huntsman for my PET scan. A PET scan is a long procedure. They escorted me back to the preparation room where they inserted an IV line. Next they injected the radioactive glucose into my body. At Huntsman they had me sit for an hour and fifteen minutes so the glucose had time to travel throughout my body. I fell asleep in the chair.

Next I needed to change into hospital clothes that had no metal for the scan. The PET scan took about thirty minutes or so. As I mentioned, it was not as bad as an MRI, not as claustrophobic.

When I was done with the scan the nurse removed the IV and sent me on my way. We had about three hours until my appointment with Dr. Canon, so Nancy drove me home and we had lunch. I had been fasting for the scan so I was hungry.

Arriving back at Huntsman, the nurse escorted us back and took my vitals. Then a student doctor came in and asked me a battery of questions. Huntsman is a training hospital so that was very common. He left and about fifteen minutes later Dr. Canon came in. He sat down and said, "Everything is looking good." To that I replied, "That is not what I want to hear. Say, 'You don't have cancer." Dr. Canon laugh and said, "You don't have cancer." Then he pulled up my PET scan image to show me that there were no "hot spots" on my full body image.

"They do want me to take a close look at your throat since there was some mucositis that inhibited the scan." So, back down my right nostril he went with a scope. The image was displayed on full color monitors that were hanging on the wall in the exam room. Nancy was fascinated to see the inside of my nasal cavity and the back of my tongue close up. For the most part, I kept my eyes closed and tried not to gag as the scope snaked down my throat.

After removing the scope, Dr. Canon followed up on the previous news by saying, "It all looks good. No signs of the tumor." Dr. Canon had been the one to scope my throat in April when we were considering whether or not I was a candidate for surgery.

After Dr. Canon was all finished with me, his nurse stayed behind to remove my feeding tube. That tube had been in me for over three months at the time. I was glad to see it go, but nervous about getting all of my nutrition via mouth. I still had some difficulty swallowing normal food. As it turned out, I would just need to be patient and take it slowly.

The official news from Dr. Canon was obviously a huge relief. I thanked God immediately. The plan to keep me cancer free was set for check-ups every 3 months for the first year. Twice a year until I reached the 5 year mark and then once a year from then on. My first quarterly check up was going to fall during the Christmas holiday so they bumped it to January 2020.

The Moral of the Story

As I complete the final chapter it has been two plus months since I got the good news. I am completely off of the pain medicine, muscle relaxers, etc. The only thing I take now is vitamins and supplements to aid my weight training routine. For the most part, I am beginning to feel like my old self again. My energy and motivation are better than they have been in months and my mental focus is more sharp.

Just as I was compiling this last bit and starting the book formatting process, a report was made public by researchers from Memorial Sloan Kettering Cancer Center and NASA recommending that cancer patients engage in a rigorous physical training regime much like NASA astronauts. Look up **"Multisystem Toxicity in Cancer: Lessons from NASA's Countermeasures Program"**. The upshot is that astronauts deal with muscle atrophy and other physical problems that are similar to those experienced by cancer patients undergoing treatment.

The medical community is doing a good job defeating the cancer cells, but the treatments; radiation and chemotherapy, leave the patient's body weak and damaged. It is that physical damage from the treatment, along with the nasty side effects that continue to harm and sometimes kill patients.

The Kettering/NASA study suggests that more research needs to be done and experience gained in order to recommend physical training. What I know from my experience is that strength training, nutrition, and faith were all tools in my fighting arsenal. You can do as you like, however, my recommendation is that you work on getting your body strong. That strength will benefit you tremendously in the fight to come.

Regardless of your situation, whether you have a cancer diagnosis, other illness, or perhaps you are just dealing with the daily demons that we all face, remember, fighting solves everything. Rather than belabor the point, let's wrap this up so that you can get yourself into the gym and start getting strong.

From Nancy

A roller coaster of emotions has been my ride through the toughest year of my life. I am a woman of faith. My feet stand on a mountain made solely of faith. What does one do when that faith is tested? Trust. Trust in God.

El Cancer did not take my husband. But if it had, I would still have my faith and my trust in God. I know God has a plan. I have lived my life believing that 100%. That belief made this entire journey through El Cancer an easier one. Oh, I had my moments. I had the kinds of moments that make others want to run as far from you as they can possibly get. Those moments of anger, disbelief, frustration, sorrow, heartache... I experienced them, but I never questioned my faith. My faith has given me the courage to be supportive to, and of, Paul. My family gave me the courage to face my own heartache, look past it, and be purely there to help Paul fight the toughest fight of his life. We fought this battle as a family. Never once did I feel alone.

I kept a journal from the time we found out about the cancer until now. It's not quite finished, as the ending will not come until Paul has passed that 5 year mark. The final journal entry will be the one saying "Paul is now cancer free." I'm looking forward to writing that one. I am including some of my journal entries here. They tell a better story than I can because they were written during the fight.

2/22/2019- 9:08am- "You want to get up and come out here so we can talk?" Crawling up from the depths of a contented sleep, I opened my bleary eyes to see my husband standing above me. "What?" I say. My mind is in a fog, I can barely open my eyes. I can't figure out why he would be standing here asking me if I want to leave my cozy bed.

I took the early shift with the dog; 6:00 am breakfast and then let out to do his business. I had lain back down shortly after 8:00 am. I hear Paul's voice again, and the words that would begin the change in our lives came tumbling out of his mouth. "The doctor called." Three little words; four little syllables. Such a short sentence. How can such a short sentence bring with it a monumental change? I don't know. "What did he say" I asked. Paul looked at me like I had lost my mind. I don't know why I asked that while I was still in bed, still bleary eyed, still wrapped in my warm, cozy blanket. I guess I already knew the answer. In my heart, I knew that Paul would not be standing, solemn, beside the bed asking me to get up and come talk, if what the doctor had to say was any different than what it actually was. Maybe I was trying to beat back the inevitable for just a few more minutes. A few more minutes of our normal life. "Well, he didn't say it wasn't" is what I heard next, then Paul turned and left the room. I quickly followed, all fog was lifted. I found Paul sitting at the kitchen table, staring into a bowl of oatmeal that he had been eating when the call came in. Gently, I asked "What did he say?" again. Paul looked at me, the weight of the world showing in his eyes. I knew. I didn't need him to say the words. I didn't need to hear the words my wonderful husband uttered next; "It's cancer."

5/11/2019 - It's been a while and a lot has happened since I last wrote. Honestly, writing this is hard and I don't want to do it, yet I do want to do it. Staring reality in the face is hard, but writing this is therapeutic, as it allows me to put my thoughts and feelings into words. I hope to write more often. One day I will look back on this and it will all be a distant memory; just a part of life that happened and we got through it. Not only got through it, but came out on the other side as better people; a better individual, a better husband and wife, a better family. I have an amazing family and I am grateful for that.

I'll start this today by saying I'm no longer angry. I was so very angry about everything for a few weeks, especially having to move over to Utah. I finally realized (by reading a Bible study passage and devotional) that I was just hanging onto, and glorifying, the past. I've always taken life in stride.

I've always been of the mind that God has a plan and wherever he takes me, I will willingly follow, even if I don't understand why. I've always gone with my heart, because I know God lives in my heart and guides me. I've always said I don't care where I live or what I'm doing, as long as I have God and my family. Most importantly, I've always believed that God takes care of us and everything will be ok. Well, what a disservice to God to be angry and bitter about having to move to Salt Lake City.

No, I don't particularly like it here, but it's not a horrible place and I was trying to find any reason I could to hate it here. There's way too many people for me. BUT, it's absolutely beautiful here. The mountains are so close and amazingly beautiful, truly a sight to behold. The tree canopy on our street is a lovely sight as I drive home. AND, I get to see Jarrad and Alex more. I missed them. How could I not appreciate such wonderful gifts from God? I'm ashamed of myself for allowing myself to be angry and bitter as I travel this path God has put before me. Never again. Even during the angry/bitter weeks, I still knew in my heart that God was with me and guiding me, holding my hand, and probably carrying me a little (more likely a lot) as well. I just needed to get myself sorted out and back on track.

I'M BACK! My heart is lighter, my eyes see more beauty, my mind is more positive. I'm thankful to God for helping me get through those rough weeks. I realize it's the circumstance and not the place itself. Salt Lake City means cancer. I'm not going to let that darken my heart.

Paul is now doing radiation therapy. He had 4 treatments this week, and next week he starts 5 treatments per week. He is scheduled into the 3rd week of June, which will be then end of his 30 treatments. After his final treatment, he will have a few weeks of feeling not so great, then he should start to return to whatever the new normal will be. I'm hoping for minimal side effects. He's already getting dry mouth and starting to lose his taste. He's also taking a very long time to eat, as it's a little harder for him to swallow being that there is a tumor on the back of his tongue. That issue will not be getting any better anytime soon because the radiation will cause burns in his throat. I'm praying for him a lot. This is going to be tough for him and it's so, so hard for me to watch him have to go through this.

We had a consultation with a chemo doctor a couple of weeks ago. The tumor board at Huntsman recommended radiation therapy with a chemo booster, which means Paul would have had the thirty radiation treatments as well as having chemo once each week, at the beginning of the week. The purpose of the chemo, which the doctor called 'chemo lite', would be to act as a booster for the radiation therapy. There was a 10-15% chance that chemo would add to the successful treatment of the cancer.

The risks were not worth the benefit to Paul. One of the biggest side effects of Cisplatin chemo is hearing loss. Paul already has a degree of hearing loss from his time in the Marine Corps. This side effect of the chemo treatments is almost guaranteed, as it is a very common side effect for those who have received Cisplatin chemotherapy. The hearing loss would be permanent. There is also the chance of neuropathy, which would also be permanent. Chemo is a poison of sorts, as it destroys your body in order to fix your body. Paul was calling the chemo doctor "Dr. Poison" before we ever had the consultation. Paul initially gave consent for the chemo treatments, but after a couple of days of thinking about it and researching Cisplatin, and agonizing over whether or not it was worth taking the chance without the chemo, Paul decided he didn't really want to do it.

We had a long, long talk in the middle of the night. Paul was torn up about getting chemo. Just the thought of having chemo was destroying him on the inside. Was a 10-15% chance of success better than not taking it? Were the doctors over treating in the interest of safety? Is there enough research to prove that Cisplatin actually does boost the radiation enough to call it a necessity? So many questions, not enough answers.

My opinion is that Paul should go with his heart, and I will support him in whatever decision he makes. It's his body and he would be the one living with side effects. I love that man with all my heart and it just killed me to have to watch him war with himself over this. He's fighting for his life. He decided against the chemo and once that burden was removed, he felt a lot better and was ready to fight.

5/16/2019 - It's been a rough week for Paul. Tomorrow will be the end of week 2 of radiation treatments. Paul has a 'yuck mouth' all the time and he's quickly losing his sense of taste. He also has an upset stomach all the time. Right now he's sleeping. He worked this morning, then worked out and when he got home he ate a little bit of cottage cheese then said he wanted to go to sleep so his stomach would quit hurting. I ordered an essential oil diffuser and some peppermint oil, as well as some peppermint oil roll ons. Hopefully that will help with the nausea. Bless his heart. Neither one of us expected the side effects to hit so quickly. We were expecting them after the 3rd week of treatments.

I went back with him to the radiation room last Friday. It was horrifying. I wanted to run. It was so uncomfortable for me to be there and I can only imagine how horrible it must be for Paul. Once he checks in, he goes back into the treatment waiting room which is down the hall from his radiation vault. He's in vault 5 each time. He changes into a hospital gown (not anymore though, as his mom made him some awesome scrub tops that he can wear. The staff loves them and I think they help Paul to feel less like a patient and more like a fighter) then he goes into his vault. Inside the vault is a huge machine with a rotating arm. Paul is put on a moveable board and has to have his head secured to the board, which is done by placing the custom radiation mask over his face. The mask looks like a net but it's hard and it's custom fitted to his face. When they made the mask, Paul had to lay there wearing it until it hardened, which took about 20 minutes. Before they put the mask on, they give Paul a mouth guard to put in his mouth, which has a handle that sticks out of the mouth hole of the mask.

I know Paul doesn't like the mask and I know it takes him a couple of minutes to fight the urge to rip it off every single time they put it on his face. He says once it's on he keeps his eyes closed. It was heartbreaking for me to watch them secure his head to the table, especially knowing how uncomfortable it is for him. I wanted to cry. Paul's radiation tech is named Dan, and Dan took the time to show me exactly what they do to get Paul ready for the radiation. He explained to me how the radiation machine works and how they line him up properly. I saw the red beams they use to line him up with the little tattoos they put on him previously. (He has 3 permanent tattoos that they circle each time he comes in. They are placed on each shoulder and the middle of his collarbone area) They also put pegs in on each side of the table for Paul to hold onto.

I felt like someone was stabbing my heart as I stood there looking at my wonderful husband on that board. I couldn't get out of there fast enough. It didn't help that on our way in we saw the Life Flight team taking someone out. It looked like that person's entire team was following down the hall to the elevator. A sad reminder of what could be.

I don't know what to do for Paul. It's hard watching him suffer. I wish it was me instead of him. Paul has never been a drinker, smoker, drug user, partier..... None of that. He doesn't deserve this. This is where our Faith comes in. No, Paul doesn't deserve it, but God knows what he is going through. We have to trust God in this and know that Paul will be ok. We have to get through the next couple of months.

5/27/2019 excerpt - I need to get some thank you card designs ready. I have so many thank you cards to write. I want to make sure to write each one of them myself. The support, love, prayers, messages, and gifts that have been sent to Paul brighten his day and warms our hearts. It's amazing how a handwritten note, or a sticker, or a book can touch ones heart so much. I'm grateful for each and every one of those things that Paul gets, as well as the messages I get.

Paul had his 2nd (and final) MRI this past week. He said he doesn't think he could do it now since he'd have to lay in the machine for at least an hour. Hopefully someday, somewhere along the way, someone will benefit from the study they are doing. We did find out that the tumor on Paul's tongue is getting smaller. The study doctor came out and talked to me while Paul was still in the MRI machine. She told me the tumor on his tongue was "liquifying", which is what it should be doing. She said he still has the tumor in his lymph node. I'm not sure what that means, but I assume the radiation will get that one too. I have no doubt this treatment will be successful.... It's just the getting through it part. I've asked God to please carry Paul the rest of the way. This is the time when there will be only one set of footprints in the sand. I can't imagine going through something like this without faith. How do people do it if they don't believe in God? Where does the strength come from? Where does the courage come from? I wouldn't know where to begin if I didn't begin with God.

6/2/2019 - The past week has been really, really rough for Paul. Paul is now in the hospital. We got Hydrocodone - Acetaminophen on Tuesday. By Thursday, the pain was so bad that those pills weren't relieving any of the pain, so the doc gave Paul Morphine pills to take as well. He was taking a morphine pill every 12 hours AND a Hydro pill, sometimes 2 pills every 4 hours. Still not relieving the pain. When the doc prescribed the morphine, we also had to get narcan in case of an accidental overdose. That's a terrifying thought.

Friday evening around 5pm was the last time he ate anything. And saying "ate" is a stretch since he has only been drinking his meals for over a week now. Saturday morning I brought him to the ER, where we spent 6 hours before he was transferred up to the Huntsman Cancer Hospital. They are giving him pain medicine for his throat every 2 hours, as well as medicine to ease his stomach pain. He's also getting constant IV fluids. They placed an NG feeding tube down his nostril today, bypassing his stomach and going straight to his intestine. The first time the nurse put anything down the tube, Paul threw it up... tube and all. It was awful. As soon as the nurse finished the medicine, Paul asked if it was normal to feel like he was going to throw up. The nurse said yes, and that the feeling would pass. About 2 seconds later, Paul was vomiting. He vomited up the tube and a shit ton of blood. It scared me half to death. In his vomiting panic, he was pulling at the feeding tube and I was terrified he would rip it out of his nose.

The nurse grabbed some scissors and cut it before he could do that. (The feeding tube was secured by a string tie of sorts that went around the back of his nostrils). Almost the entire length of the feeding tube came out when Paul was vomiting. I doubt I'll ever forget the sight of him hunched over, feeding tube hanging out of his mouth, blood pouring out. I thought something had torn as the tube came back up. The nurse said the blood was just from the irritation in his throat. After the nurse removed the tied part of the tube from his nose, Paul was able to rinse his mouth out and brush his teeth. He seems ok now, but that doesn't fix the fact that he has not eaten in well over 48 hours. I think he will have to get the peg tube for feeding.

The devil is trying to get us. A "spiritual volunteer" stopped in today and asked if we would like to attend a service or have a visit from the Chaplain. Paul asked that the Chaplain stop by for a prayer and communion. Jarrad and Zach also participated in communion. Since then, it's just been a rough day all around. That doesn't change the fact that we are standing on our Faith. Clearly the devil is trying to drive a wedge in that foundation of faith. It isn't going to work. No matter what happens, we will still have our Faith.

Last night was a nightmare for Paul. I was hoping that since he was being given enough pain medicine to ease his pain that he would be able to sleep. That's impossible in this place. There's always a monitor beeping or someone coming in to take blood or vitals or change a bag or check on Paul. Paul's pulse drops so low when they give him the pain meds that it sets off the alarm every couple of minutes. Once it drops down below 40, the alarm rings. When they give Paul the pain medicine, his pulse runs between 35 & 40 for about 45 minutes. The nurse finally turned the volume down today after Paul said he couldn't take another night of that mess. I understand he needs the alarm, but he also needs to rest.

It's 11:00pm on Sunday. At the moment Paul is sleeping. The nurse gave him some pain med and some ativan. I hope he sleeps for most of the night.

I'm scared. I guess it's ok to admit that. I'm scared and I feel helpless. The radiation is killing the cancer, but is it also killing Paul? His body has had such a tough time from the beginning. Neither one of us expected him to have such a hard time. Paul was told that the radiation would feel like having a sunburn in his throat. That is so far from the truth that someone needs to be slapped for telling such a big lie. Poor Paul. He said every time he tries to swallow something, even a drink of water, that it feels like someone is jamming an ice pick down his throat. One of the speech and swallow therapists told us today that head and neck cancer radiation is so horrible for people that if she was diagnosed with the same cancer that she would not get the treatment. And she sees this all the time. I can only imagine how horrible this must be for Paul.

People are praying and I am so thankful for that. We need the prayer.

6/6/2019 - They make it sound so easy; 30 radiation treatments, it will feel like a sunburn in your throat, you'll have a hard time swallowing, you may or may not lose some hair, etc. This is not easy. Paul's body is taking a beating right now. Everything makes him sick, everything causes him pain. I can't even imagine how he must feel right now. After today's radiation, he will have 8 more treatments. We are so close to the end of this mess. I hope Paul can keep that fighting spirit going for a few more weeks. I'm so glad now that he chose not to do the chemo. I'm not sure how well he would fare had he done so. I talked to another patient's wife yesterday. Her husband has throat cancer as well and is in the ICU right now. He has done 10 radiation treatments and 3 chemo treatments and she said he has been so sick since the start of treatment. He got an infection in his gall bladder and it burst. She said the chemo is making him so sick that he has already lost 40lbs....weight he could not afford to lose. Hearing her story makes me even more glad that Paul chose not to have chemo.

As the day has progressed, Paul seems to be doing a little better. We were hoping to get home today, but that changed this morning and now we will hope to get home tomorrow. Tomorrow will be a week that Paul has been in this hospital. After radiation this morning Paul got very sick and threw up. The nurse finally figured it out. They changed his pain medicine yesterday and it was not agreeing with him. The doc has stopped the hydrocodone and will be moving him to a pill form of the one pain med that isn't making him loopy as hell or sick to his stomach. I hope that works well for him. I did a couple of tube feeds for Paul today and so far he has been able to keep it down and there are no complications to deal with now. He is supposed to have 240cc's of the blended food each time he is fed. So far he has been able to take 120cc's. Next time we feed him we will be trying 180cc's. Let's hope this works well so he can get home.

6/13/2019 - 3 more radiation treatments to go. Paul was finally released from the hospital this past

Saturday afternoon. We thought he would get to go home on Friday, but he was still a bit dehydrated, so they gave him more IV fluid and kept him another day. I'm so glad his pain is finally under control. He now wears a 50mcg fentanyl patch that we change every 72 hours. He also takes 4mg dilaudid every 4 hours for breakthrough pain, except at night when he takes 8mg so he can go a little more than 4 hours. And we still have the Narcan in case of an accidental overdose, which is more of a threat to us now because of the patch. I have to make sure to wear gloves when removing the old patch and placing the new one.

I've been doing blenderized tube feedings for him and so far he has tolerated those well. It's just hard to get him enough calories and 2L of fluid each day because his stomach has shrunk so much. I created a more calorie dense base meal today, so that should help. Our first night home I managed to get the feeding tube clogged. What a kick in the arse that was. Scared me half to death. We used Coke as the nurse suggested when she was going over the feeding procedures with us. Of course, that did not work. So Paul suggested a thin piece of wire. I found one and Paul managed to get the tube cleared. Thank The Lord! I hope that never happens again. I sure don't want to have to go back to the hospital to have them unclog the tube or replace the tube.

Dr. H is out of the office this week, so on our normal Wednesday visit we saw a different doc and Rebecca (Dr. H's nurse). The visit went well. Paul has lost right around 22lbs since starting radiation. That's not too bad, but he's looking pretty thin in the face. At the very end of the visit, Rebecca surprised me by telling us that every now and then a patient comes along and proves them wrong. She said Paul is that patient right now. She talked about how Paul had such severe reactions to the radiation, which is not normally the case. She said he's had such a hard time and has had side effects others do not, and how hard this treatment has been on his body.

Everyone is different and the "standard" side effects are the norm. Paul is way outside the realm of the norm. It was nice to hear her admit that they were wrong to tell Paul he needed to toughen up and that he didn't need the feeding tube, he just needed to force himself to swallow food and fluid. (That's what Dr. H told him) Rebecca also gave Paul some burn cream for his neck because his neck looks like he's got a terrible burn. Hopefully the cream will start healing the skin faster than aloe has been. I've been putting the cream on twice per day and his neck looks better already.

7/15/2019 - It's been almost a month since Paul has finished his radiation. He's not healed yet. He still has the radiation burns, the feeding tube, the fatigue, the pain meds. Paul is getting discouraged because he feels like his body should be all healed up now. Apparently it's a much slower process than we were expecting. Maybe because Paul had such a hard time with the radiation itself. Looking back on what we were told way back at the beginning, versus the reality.... I realize how different those two stories really are. Paul is healing and will continue to do so. We have to wait until September for Paul to have another PET scan to make sure the cancer is gone. Seems like a long time, doesn't it? Emotional torture, followed by physical torture, followed by more emotional torture. Living the dream.

I sound cynical, don't I? I shouldn't be. I'm thankful. Thankful for the hope treatment has brought us. I'm thankful for my faith. I'm thankful for my family and my Grad program family. I'm thankful for our friends. I'm thankful for the strangers who took the time to send encouraging words. I'm thankful for so many things. As the saying goes, time heals all wounds. Patience has never been my strong suit :)

8/29/2019 - Paul and I are going to Saratoga this weekend. Leaving tomorrow and coming back on Sunday. We are going to stay out at Elk Hollow. I just wanted to give Paul a couple days of peace. He has missed this entire year of being able to tromp around the outdoors...something he absolutely loves to do. No prairie dogs this year... no climbing the mountains... no days spent on the range. I hope this weekend will do his soul some good. On Saturday Paul is going out shooting with an old friend of his. It'll be nice for Paul to spend a little time with someone who thinks like he does :)

9/11/2019 - Paul is cancer free! Thank God. I didn't realize how scared Paul had been until we were in the hallway after the appointment and Paul said if he didn't get out of there he was going to start crying right there. What a relief that must have been for him. After all that fear, pain, emotional and physical torment... to finally know it was all worth it.

11/11/2019 - The last 2 months have been spent dealing with weaning off the opioid meds and the withdrawal that comes along with that process. We thought when Paul found out he was cancer free that the best was to come. Boy were we wrong. Don't get me wrong...cancer free is a huge blessing and we are thankful for that. Watching Paul suffer through the withdrawal was heartbreaking. Hasn't he suffered enough? The radiation pain, the tube feedings, the infections, the cancer itself, weren't those enough?? Apparently not. Withdrawal was yet to come. The sleepless nights, foggy brain, muscle aches, the pain of his body being physically addicted to medicine that he had to have at one point but no longer needs. The body doesn't understand that though... doesn't understand that it does not need the medicine.

Paul suffered through the withdrawal for weeks. It would have been so easy to just take another pill and make it all go away. His body wanted that pill but his mind did not. One final battle. The struggle between the mind and the body. The mind knows what the body does not. Physical or mental... which one wins? In this case, the mind finally won. The physical addiction has finally passed. Paul is no longer afraid to go to sleep. He knows he can sleep now. He knows he will no longer wake up feeling a pain he can do nothing about. The pain clinic gave him a muscle relaxer to "help" with the muscle aches. It did absolutely nothing to alleviate the pain. Maybe that med works on some people, but it sure didn't work on Paul. I can totally see why people choose to stay on opioids for years and years.

Paul doesn't go back to see a doctor until January. He will have to be seen every 3 months for the first year. They won't officially declare him "cancer free" until he has been 5 years past the most recent PET scan. See you in 5 years to say "Paul is cancer free"!

Paul ran straight into the cancer fight, head held high, doing what had to be done despite the fear and uncertainty. He's braver than I would have been. I hope he knows how brave I think he is.

God has been good to us. We have had a very rough year. Here we are now, nearing the end of the worst year of our lives, knowing that when we start the next year we will be doing so with all of this mess behind us. The light is bright. God has been so good to us.

Recipes for Fighters
(through the tube)

Blended Meal Base #1

3 oz Carrots, Frozen
2 oz Broccoli, Frozen
2.75 oz Cauliflower, Frozen
2 oz No Sugar Added Raspberries, Frozen
4 oz Chicken Broth
8.5 oz Canned Chicken Breast
2 Servings Keto Greens Powder, Lemon Flavor
1 Serving Fitness Fiber Powder
1 Serving Organic Spirulina Powder

Yield 8 Servings

Per Serving Nutrition -
50.5 Calories
4.0g Carbohydrates
2.2g Fiber
1.8g Net Carbs
1.2g Sugar
6.1g Protein
1.7g Fat
19.0mg Cholesterol
0.3 Glycemic Load

Blended Meal Base #2

16 oz Ground Turkey 85% Lean
.5 c Chicken Bone Broth
3 oz Cauliflower, Frozen
3 oz Broccoli, Frozen
3 oz Carrots, Frozen

Yield 8 Servings

Per Serving Nutrition -
122.8 Calories
1.8g Carbohydrates
1.0g Fiber
0.8g Net Carbohydrates
0.7g Sugar
10.7g Protein
8.7g Fat
48.1mg Cholesterol
0.4 Glycemic Load

Blended Meal Base #3

1 c Chicken Bone Broth
3 oz Carrots, Frozen
3 oz Spinach, Frozen
2 oz Broccoli, Frozen
3 oz Cauliflower, Frozen
3 oz Beef Chuck Roast
3.33 oz Chicken (Light and Dark meat)
5 Links Maple Sausage
6 Slices Bacon
.25 c Organic Extra Virgin Olive Oil
2 Servings Keto Micro Greens Powder, Lemon Flavor
6 Tbsp Ranch Dressing
3 Servings Tahini

Yields 10 Servings

Per Serving Nutrition -
257.5 Calories
4.6g Carbohydrates
2.1g Fiber
2.5g Net Carbs
1.4g Sugar
11.7g Protein
22.4g Fat
25.9mg Cholesterol
0.4 Glycemic Load

Blended Meal Base #4

4.37 oz Summer Squash, Fresh
3.03 oz Zucchini, Fresh
.25 c Chicken Bone Broth
4.16 oz Chicken Breast
1 Slice Beef Liver (3.99oz)
3 Pork Sausage Links
8 oz Milked Walnuts, Unsweetened
6 Tbsp Organic Extra Virgin Olive Oil
2 Servings SWAT Fuel Protein Powder
6 Tbsp Ranch Dressing

Yields 10 Servings

Per Serving Nutrition -
207.6 Calories
2.6g Carbohydrates
0.3g Fiber
2.3g Net Carbohydrates
0.8g Sugar
13.2g Protein
16.5g Fat
56.2mg Cholesterol
0.3 Glycemic Load

Blended Meal Base #5

16oz Breakfast Sausage
2 Tbsp Olive Oil
3.5 oz Organic Chopped Kale, Frozen
3.5 oz Organic Chopped Spinach, Frozen
1 C Organic Chicken Bone Broth
6 oz Cauliflower, Frozen
1 C Walnut Milk
.75 C Ranch Salad Dressing
8 tsp Unflavored Fitness Fiber

Yields 10 Servings

Per Serving Nutrition -
323.8 Calories
8.5g Carbohydrates
5.0g Fiber
3.5g Net Carbohydrates
0.4g Sugar
8.5g Protein
29.7g Fat
36.4mg Cholesterol
0.2 Glycemic Load

Blended Meal Base #6

6 oz Chopped Spinach, Frozen
5 oz Chopped Kale, Frozen
7 oz Pumpkin, Frozen
15 oz Can Whole New Potatoes
2 Tbsp Olive Oil
6 Tbsp MCT Oil
.67 C Ranch Salad Dressing
16 oz Small Shrimp, no tails, Frozen

Yields 10 Servings

Per Serving Nutrition -
252.4 Calories
7.8g Carbohydrates
1.3g Fiber
6.5g Net Carbohydrates
0.6g Sugar
12.5g Protein
19.0g Fat
97.2mg Cholesterol
0.1 Glycemic Load

Blended Meal Base #7

16 oz Ground Turkey, Festive Brand
12 oz Small Shrimp, no tails, Frozen
1 Can Corned Beef Hash
15 oz Can Whole New Potatoes
4 Servings Keto Microgreens Powder, Lemon
2 C Chicken Bone Broth
8 Tbsp Olive Oil
8 Tbsp Ranch Salad Dressing

Yields 14 Servings

Per Serving Nutrition -
256.3 Calories
6.2g Carbohydrates
0.9g Fiber
5.3g Net Carbohydrates
0.4g Sugar
10.7g Protein
20.7g Fat
66.1mg Cholesterol
0.1 Glycemic Load

Blended Meal Base #8

16 oz Wild Caught Cod
16 oz All Natural Turkey Sausage
10.5 oz Spinach, Frozen
2 C Chicken Bone Broth
8 Tbsp Olive Oil
4 Tbsp MCT Oil
1.5 C Whole Milk Plain Greek Yogurt

Yields 14 Servings

Per Serving Nutrition -
216.8 Calories
2.3g Carbohydrates
0.8g Fiber
1.5g Net Carbohydrates
1.1g Sugar
15.7g Protein
16.3g Fat
48.0mg Cholesterol
0.1 Glycemic Load

Keto Recipes (through the mouth)

Lemon Lime Fat Bombs
20 Servings

8oz Philadelphia Brand Original Cream Cheese, softened
5 Tbsp Butter
1 Tbsp Lemon Juice
1 Tbsp Lime Juice
1 tsp Lemon Zest
3 Tbsp Lakanto Classic Monkfruit Sweetener

You'll need to make sure your cream cheese and butter are softened but not melted. Either let both sit on the counter for about an hour, or simply heat in microwave for about 30 seconds, which is what I do.

In a stand mixer (if you don't have one, a hand mixer works as well) blend cream cheese and butter until well mixed. Add lemon juice, lime juice, lemon zest, and sweetener. Mix on medium speed for 5-7 minutes. Mixture should be well blended and you should not have any cream cheese chunks left.

While your mixer is running, either prepare your fat bomb molds or line a glass dish with parchment paper. I use a 7.5x5.5 dish and it easily makes 20 good sized fat bombs.

Once ingredients are well mixed and there are no lumps of cream cheese left, transfer mix to your molds or dish. Place in freezer for 2 hours, then transfer to refrigerator. You can freeze extra batches for a couple of weeks if you make extra. Once the fat bombs are placed in the refrigerator, you will need to eat them within 7 days. (Not a problem! They are delicious)

Each Serving Contains -
67 Calories
.8 g Protein
6.8 g Fat
2.3 g Total Carbs
0 g Fiber
1.8 g Sugar Alcohols
.5 g Net Carbs

Keto Pizza Crust (tastes like REAL pizza crust)
12 servings, Serving Size: 1/12 slice (dough only)

1 C almond meal (or almond flour)
½ tsp garlic salt
½ tsp Italian seasoning
½ tsp pizza crust yeast
1 and ¾ cups shredded mozzarella cheese
2 tablespoons cream cheese
1 egg

Preheat oven to 425°F

In a small bowl, mix together dry ingredients.

In a larger, microwavable bowl, mix together the mozzarella cheese and cream cheese. Microwave for 1 minute. Remove from microwave and stir until mixed. Microwave for an additional 15 seconds.

Add dry ingredients to cheese mixture, blend well. This gives the cheese a little time to cool before adding the egg.

Add egg, blend well. You should have a slightly sticky ball of dough once all ingredients are well mixed. (I mixed with my very clean hands)

Place dough ball on a piece of parchment paper and hand flatten the dough ball. Cover with another piece of parchment paper and use a rolling pin to roll out the dough. I baked on a rectangle stone pan, so my dough was rolled out in a rectangle, and I rolled it pretty thin so the crust was a little thinner than a normal pizza crust. If you like a thick crust pizza, you'll need to cook the crust a little longer.

Bake crust for 12-15 minutes. Add sauce and desired pizza toppings and bake for an additional 5-10 minutes ...just long enough to warm toppings and melt the cheese.

Each Serving Contains -
102.5 Calories
6.2 g Protein
7.8 g Fat
2.7 g Total Carbs
1.0 g Fiber
1.7 g Net Carbs

Keto Veggie Pizza
12 Servings

1 Keto Pizza Dough

8 ounces (about half a can of the Muir) Organic Pizza Sauce (the organic usually has less carbs. I used Muir Glen)

1 - 8 ounce Fresh Mozzarella Cheese Ball

1 Cup Shredded Mozzarella Cheese

2 ounce Tomato (I use either grape or cherry tomatoes and cut them in half)

⅔ ounce Diced Green Bell Pepper

1 ounce Red Bell Peppers, Raw

¾ ounce Sweet Cherry Peppers by Mezzetta

1-½ ounce Artichoke Hearts or Quarters, Canned In Oil Mixture

Bake pizza dough as directed in Keto Pizza Dough Recipe. Evenly spread the pizza sauce over the pre cooked dough. Slice the mozzarella cheese ball and spread slices evenly over pizza dough. I try to cut my mozzarella cheese about ¼" thick. Sprinkle all veggie ingredients on top of mozz cheese, spreading as evenly as possible.

Sprinkle shredded mozz cheese over veggies and bake at 350℉ for 10-15 minutes... long enough for the cheese to melt and the veggies to warm.
If you use different or more/less than what is in this recipe, your nutrition information changes. If you use the Carb Manager app, you can put all the ingredients in a recipe and it will give you the nutrition information.

Each Serving Contains -
197.4 Calories
12.3 g Protein
13.9 g Fat
6.5 g Total Carbs
1.6 g Fiber
4.8 g Net Carbs

Keto Meat Pizza

12 Servings

1 Keto Pizza Dough

8 ounces (about half a can of the Muir) Organic Pizza Sauce (the organic usually has less carbs. I used Muir Glen)

1 1/2 Cups Shredded Mozzarella Cheese

2/3 Cup Shredded Colby Jack Cheese

3 1/2 ounces Grass Fed Ground Beef, browned.

3 ounces Pepperoni Slices

2 ounce Tomato (I use either grape or cherry tomatoes and cut them in half)

3/4 ounce Diced Green Bell Pepper

Bake pizza dough as directed in Keto Pizza Dough Recipe. Evenly spread the pizza sauce over the pre cooked dough. Sprinkle shredded mozz cheese over the sauce as evenly as possible. Lay pepperonis evenly over mozz cheese. Sprinkle browned ground beef over pepperoni. Add veggie ingredients on top of meats, spreading as evenly as possible. Sprinkle shredded colby jack cheese over veggies and bake at 350°F for 10-15 minutes... long enough for the cheese to melt and the veggies to warm.

If you use different or more/less than what is in this recipe, your nutrition information changes. If you use the Carb Manager app, you can put all the ingredients in a recipe and it will give you the nutrition information.

Each Serving Contains -
238.0 Calories
14.1 g Protein
18.2 g Fat
5.3 g Total Carbs
1.4 g Fiber
3.9 g Net Carbs

Keto Chili
12 Servings

2.5 lbs Grass Fed Ground Beef
1 28oz Can Organic Diced Tomatoes
1 28oz Can Organic Crushed Tomatoes
5oz Mushrooms
3 Cloves Fresh Garlic, minced
1 Small Green Bell Pepper, diced
5 tsp Chili Powder
1 tsp Cumin, ground
1 tsp Sea Salt
1 tsp Black Pepper
1 tsp Onion Powder
½ tsp Crushed Red Pepper Flakes
½ tsp Smoked Paprika
1 ½ C Chicken Bone Broth

Brown Ground Beef in large soup pot. Once beef is cooked, add garlic, mushrooms and bell pepper. Saute for 15 minutes, stirring frequently. Add all dry seasonings and stir well. Once seasonings are thoroughly mixed with meat and veggies, reduce heat to low and add both cans of tomatoes. Stir well, then add bone broth. Allow to simmer for 2 -3 hours. If using a crock pot, once the meat is browned, veggies are sauteed and dry seasonings are added, everything can be put in the crock pot and cooked on low for 6-8 hours.

Each Serving Contains -
233 Calories
19.5 g Protein
13.1 g Fat
9 g Total Carbs
3.4 g Fiber
5.6 g Net Carbs Per Serving

Keto Lemon Cheesecake
8 Servings

Preheat oven to 350°F

Crust
6 Tbsp Butter
2 C Almond Meal
⅓ C Lakanto Classic Monkfruit Sweetener
1 Tbsp Lemon Zest

Mix all dry ingredients together until well mixed. Add butter and mix well. (I use my very clean hands)
Once all mixed, spread into a round, deep dish baking pan, running the mix up the sides of pan to edge.
Bake at 350 for 15 minutes, then remove from oven and let cool for about 5 minutes. Reduce oven temp to 325°F.

While the crust is baking, mix up cheesecake.

Lemon Cheesecake

2 8oz Packages Philadelphia Original Cream Cheese
2 Eggs
1 C Lakanto Classic Monkfruit Sweetener
1 tsp vanilla extract
2 Tbsp Lemon Juice
1 Tbsp Lemon Zest

Soften cream cheese for 30 seconds in microwave. Mix all ingredients well, using a stand mixer if you have one. If not, a hand held mixer will work. (I throw it all in the bowl together)
Pour cheesecake mix into prepared crust.
Bake at 325 for 55 minutes. The cheesecake will be a little jiggly but not wet when it is completely baked.
Cool in fridge for at least 2 hours before serving. This will allow the cheesecake to properly set.
Add Lemon Whipped Cream to top of cheesecake before serving.

Lemony Whipped Cream Topping

1 C Heavy Whipping Cream
¼ C Powdered Lakanto Classic Monkfruit Sweetener (I grind the regular using a coffee grinder)
2 Tbsp Lemon Juice
1 Tbsp Lemon Zest

Blend all ingredients in a stand mixer (or hand held) until stiff peaks form. Don't overmix. The whipped cream will be thick and fluffy.... And oh so delicious!

Each Serving Contains -
524 Calories
12.3 g Protein
48 g Fat
37.7 g Total Carbs
4.3 g Fiber
26 g Sugar Alcohol
7.4 g Net Carbs

Keto Garlic Rolls

12 Rolls

2 C Almond Flour
1.5 tsp Baking Powder
.5 tsp Garlic Powder
.5 tsp Sea Salt
1 C Shredded Mozzarella Cheese
3 Tbsp Butter
.5 C Hot Water
Garlic for topping
Grated Parmesan Cheese for topping
Dried Parsley Flakes for topping

Preheat oven to 400°F
Have baking pan ready and lined with parchment paper.

In a large mixing bowl, mix together all dry ingredients except for .5 tsp garlic powder. Set aside.
In a small microwave safe bowl, melt mozzarella cheese and butter for 30 seconds. If not thoroughly melted, microwave in 15 second increments until melted.
Once cheese and butter are melted, mix together.
Add melted cheese and butter to bowl of dry ingredients. Mix well. (I use my very clean hands)
Add hot water. Mix well.

Form dough into roll shape. Dough will be sticky so you'll need to have cold water for coating your hands in order to shape the dough.

Once all rolls are formed and on the baking pan, sprinkle rolls with remaining garlic powder, grated parmesan cheese, and parsley flakes. Bake at 400°F for 12-15 minutes. Let sit for a couple of minutes before serving.

Each Serving Contains -
202.7 Calories
8.3 g Protein
17.6 g Fat
5.4 g Total Carbs
2.5 g Fiber
2.9 g Net Carbs Per Serving

Keto Cheeseburger Soup

12 Servings

1 ½ lb Grass Fed Ground Beef
2 ⅔ C Normandy Blend Frozen Vegetables
4 C Chicken Broth
4 C Water
1 14 ½ oz Can Diced Tomatoes w/ Green Chiles
1 tsp Sea Salt
1 tsp Black Pepper
1 Tbsp Italian Seasoning
¼ C Shredded Cheddar Cheese for Topping Each Serving of Soup

In large pot, brown ground beef. Once meat is brown, add sea salt, pepper and Italian seasoning. Sautee for 5 minutes to blend spices with meat. Leave any grease in the pan.
Add tomatoes w/ green chiles and mix well. Add chicken broth and water, mix well, then add veggies. Simmer on low heat for at least 1 hour. Serve soup topped with shredded cheese.

Each Serving Contains -
241 Calories
18.2 g Protein
16.7 g Fat
3.9 g Total Carbs
1 g Fiber
2.9 g Net Carbs

Keto Coconut Cream Pie
8 Servings

Crust
1/2 C Melted Butter
1 C Finely Ground Almond Flour
2 Eggs
1/4 C Sugar Substitute
1 C Coconut Flour

Melt butter in a small bowl.
In a large bowl, mix together almond flour, coconut flour, sugar substitute. Make sure to mix well.
Add eggs and butter to dry mixture. Mix well until dough forms.
Press dough into greased pie pan using your very clean fingers to spread dough into shell form.
With a fork, poke small holes around the bottom of crust.
Bake crust at 400°F for 10 minutes. Allow crust to cool.

Filling
1 C Unsweetened Coconut Flakes
1 ½ C Heavy Whipping Cream
1 ½ C Coconut Milk
1 tsp Vanilla Extract
1 tsp Xanthan Gum
2 Eggs
3/4 C Sugar Substitute
¼ tsp Salt

Spread coconut evenly on a baking sheet. Bake at 350, stirring occasionally, until golden brown, for 5-8 minutes.

In a medium saucepan, combine the heavy whipping cream, coconut milk, eggs, sugar sub, xanthan gum, salt, and vanilla extract. Mix well. Bring to a boil over low heat, stirring constantly. Cook, stirring constantly, for 2 additional minutes. (Mixture should have the consistency of custard or pudding.) Remove pan from heat, stir in ¾ C toasted coconut. Use the remaining ¼ C coconut to top the pie.

Pour the filling into the pie shell and chill until firm, 3-4 hours.

Keto Coconut Cream Pie Continued

Topping:
1 C Heavy Cream
¼ C Sugar Substitute, powdered
1 tsp Vanilla Extract

If you have a stand mixer, add all ingredients to mixing bowl and beat on medium speed until stiff peaks form. This usually takes 3-5 minutes.
If you have a hand mixer, add all ingredients to bowl and mix on low speed until stiff peaks form. If you can mix on medium speed without flinging whipped cream all over your kitchen, feel free. If using a hand mixer, this will take 3-8 minutes, depending on the speed setting.
**A reminder - If you mix the cream for too long past the peaks forming, you'll end up making butter instead of whipped cream.
Once pie has cooled for 3-4 hours, top with whipped topping and remaining coconut.

Each Serving Contains -
744.2 Calories
11.9 g Protein
67.2 g Fat
42.8 g Total Carbs
6.3 g Fiber
30 g Sugar Alcohol
6.5 g Net Carbs

Gumbo Keto and Kosher
8 servings

6 Tbsp Organic Olive Oil
5 stalks organic celery, chopped
2 bell peppers, chopped
2 tsp onion powder
½ C Organic Bone Broth Chicken
2 Chicken breast, cooked and cut into small pieces
1 Lb Turkey Chorizo
2 Cloves Fresh Garlic, finely chopped
1 Tbsp Herbs De Provence
1 tsp salt
1 tsp pepper
2 C Chicken Bone Broth
4 C water
1 28oz Can Organic Diced Tomatoes
12 oz bag frozen okra
1 Organic Bay leaf
Optional ingredient (**NOT Kosher**) - 1 lb small, cooked shrimp, tails removed. If adding shrimp, add along with the chicken

Saute celery, peppers, onion powder in 2 Tbsp olive oil
In a large soup pot, add 2 Tbsp olive Oil, Turkey Chorizo, Herbs De Provence, salt, pepper, and chopped garlic, cook well
While Turkey Chorizo mix is cooking, thoroughly cook chicken breast in 2 Tbsp olive oil and ½ C chicken bone broth

Once chicken breast is completely cooked, cut and add to soup pot of chorizo mix.

Add sauteed vegetables, diced tomatoes, and okra to soup pot. Stir ingredients together.

Add Chicken Bone Broth and Water to pot, mix ingredients together.

Crumble Bay Leaf into gumbo mixture and stir well.

Cook on low heat for 2-3 hours, until mixture is fully cooked and thickens. The okra will act as the thickener, so there's no need to add flour, cream, or file to the gumbo mix.

Each Serving Contains - **NO SHRIMP Option**
337.7 Calories
26.8 g Protein
20 g Fat
10.4 g Total Carbs
2.9 g Fiber
7.5 g Net Carbs

Keto BBQ Sauce

16 Servings - Serving Size 1 Tbsp

1 6oz Can Organic Tomato Paste
½ C Organic Apple Cider Vinegar
½ C Water
2 Tbsp Butter
½ tsp Liquid Smoke
⅓ C Powdered Golden Lakanto Monkfruit Sweetener (Grind granulated in coffee grinder to get powdered)
2 tsp Garlic Salt
1 tsp Onion Powder
1 tsp Yellow Mustard Powder
½ tsp Paprika

* If you use Smoked Paprika, eliminate the Liquid Smoke

Combine all ingredients in a small saucepan. Cover and simmer on low heat for 30 minutes. Allow to cool slightly before putting in container. Keep refrigerated. Makes approximately 8oz of sauce.

Each Serving Contains -
25 Calories
.4 g Protein
1.5 g Fat
5.9 g Total Carbs
.7 g Fiber
4 g Sugar Alcohols
1.2 g Net Carbs

A Lagniappe from Ms Nancy

When doing the blended tube feedings at home, I made sure that every single thing I put in that blender provided some type of nutritional benefit to Paul. Nothing went in his food that didn't serve a purpose, and nothing contained any type of soy product. One of the best things about eating a keto diet is that there is no soy in any of the food you eat. Paul has some food allergies and soy happens to be a big one. All of the recipes the hospital dietary specialist gave me had some type of food item that Paul was allergic to, so I had to create my own recipes.

In addition to the blended meal base I made, I added a SWAT Fuel 40 Caliber Multivitamin, Grass Fed Pure Whey Protein Powder, Fitness Fiber Powder, Broccoli Sprout Extract, Kyolic Aged Garlic Extract, Perfect Keto Micros (microgreens), Calcium Citrate, Dried Parsley, Dried Oregano, Organic Extra Virgin Olive Oil, Organic MCT Oil, Vitamin E capsules, Fish Oil capsules, Organic Spirulina Powder, Organic Goji Berry Powder, and an Organic Berry Blend powder.

Each of those items was used daily, in addition to the blended meal base. Some items I used every single meal; Olive Oil, Parsley, Oregano, Protein Powder, and Keto Greens. Most items were added to meals twice each day; Fitness Fiber, Broccoli

Sprout Extract, Kyolic Aged Garlic Extract, Organic Goji Berry Powder, and an Organic Berry Blend powder. Some items were used only for the first meal of the day; Calcium Citrate, Organic MCT Oil, Vitamin E capsules, Fish Oil capsules, and Organic Spirulina Powder. The SWAT Fuel Multivitamin was added to three meals each day. I used Organic Chicken Bone Broth instead of water to thin out the base and the additional ingredients enough to put in the feeding tube.

For hydration purposes, I only used alkaline water. A dear friend educated me on the merits of alkaline water and suggested that I use that rather than regular water for Paul. I also got some electrolyte mix to add to that alkaline water to make sure Paul was properly hydrated. Dr. Price's electrolyte mix worked great for us. I chose this specific product because it is sweetened with Stevia rather than sugar.

All of the above items can be found online. SWATFuel.com for the vitamins. They also have a great protein powder. A few items I was able to get from the local grocery, but most items came from Amazon simply because it was easier for me to have it delivered to the house. There wasn't enough time in the day to go from store to store to purchase what was needed.

There were items we used for the tube feedings that I was able to get online as well. All from Amazon. The syringes, which were much, much cheaper than the options offered by the hospital, worked perfectly. They were individually wrapped, easy glide catheter tip, 60cc, disposable syringes made by Global Medical Products. I used these syringes the entire time we had to use the feeding tube and never had a problem. I would definitely use them again if I had to. I was also able to find a belt that went around Paul's waist to secure the feeding tube. When we came home from the hospital, we were given a roll of medical tape so we could tape the hanging tube to Paul's chest. It didn't take long for us to realize how painful that was going to be for Paul because the tape irritated his skin. Everytime we had to pull the tape off his skin in order to use the tube, we left a new red mark where the tape had pulled skin with it. Core Products has a belt with a pouch on the front called a Core Products NelMed G-Tube Holder. This worked perfectly. My advice would be to go ahead and buy the two pack instead of just one. If you have a feeding tube, or need to feed someone via a tube, you know there is drainage around the tube site for the first few weeks while the skin is healing. When we came home from the hospital, they sent a type of gauze pad to put around the tube to protect the skin from the drainage. Those were fine except for the fact that the gauze would get wet due to the drainage and rub against Paul's skin, which was irritating to him. I was able to find a reusable, thicker, organic cotton padding that worked out much better than simple gauze pads. The company that makes the cotton pads is called Ian's Choice and they come in a 12 pack. Well worth it. There's always extra on hand and I was able to machine wash and dry them with no issues.

Made in the USA
Middletown, DE
12 February 2020